Lose Your Weight Naturally

Table of Contents

Chapter 1

Why do people become fat?

The standard reason given for individuals getting fat is that they eat an excessive amount of and/or exercise too little. That reflects one of the fundamental laws of thermodynamics—I overlook which one. The measure of vitality you put into a framework short the vitality you take out must be put away some place i.e. FAT! This plan—genuine however it is—does not by any means clarify obesity since a few individuals appear to eat more than fat individuals and exercise close to these same fat individuals, but they are not fat! Crediting this to the general perversity of the universe is not adequate clarification. Different components must become possibly the most important factor. I specify beneath a portion of the thoughts mindful individuals have proposed to clarify why fat individuals get to be fat:

1. It is felt that a few individuals are bound to put on weight in light of the fact that they have acquired "fat qualities" from their guardians. There can be probably individuals shift in their hereditary cosmetics and a few individuals are slanted due to hereditary motivations to end up tall, or expansive bore or squat or fat. It is known, for case that stature is controlled by various diverse qualities, likely around twenty. By the by, tallness is influenced likewise by eating routine. Fat individuals tend to originate from fat families. That doesn't inexorably imply that they are fat for hereditary reasons. They could have learned fat-production practices, i.e. dietary patterns, from their guardians when they were growing up. On account of investigations of indistinguishable twins isolated during childbirth, nonetheless, it can be said, unquestionably, that there is, in fact, a solid hereditary segment to body weight. This is not to say that somebody so developed hereditarily is bound to getting to be fat.

I once saw a lady in her mid-forties who ought to have been fat, however wasn't. She had two siblings, each of whom weighed more than four hundred pounds; and she had a developed kid who weighed more than three hundred and fifty pounds. Doubtlessly, she had whatever qualities it took to get fat. Thus, I asked her one day, "Why you're not fat?" She clarified that she thought it needed to do with the way that she kept running for 60 minutes and an a large portion of consistently before she went to the exercise center.

2. Diet. Keep in mind that law of thermodynamics. The measure of vitality that goes into a machine (the human body, for example) needs to adjust the sum that goes out; or the additional vitality that goes in (nourishment) must be put away by one means or another (fat.) So, for everybody, regardless of what that individual's hereditary weakness, either bringing down the nutrition allow or expanding the vitality

yield (exercise) will bring down the vitality put away as fat. Eating less and less or practicing more will bring about weight reduction. Our cutting edge diet is by all accounts intended to pack however many calories as could be expected under the circumstances inside of the human ability to eat. High caloric nourishments appear to be naturally more appealing than different nutritions for reasons that presumably need to do with survival in conditions that people wound up in more often than not all through our history. Be that as it may, no more.

A few cases: Chinese who lived in China subsisted on a generally calorie less than stellar eating routine and were, generally, thin and solid. Their youngsters, once they resulted in these present circumstances nation and started eating like whatever is left of the Americans, got to be fat in higher numbers and started building up each one of those ailments connected with obesity.

There is an Indian tribe that lives in a bone-dry part of the West and has lived there for some eras. (Obviously their property was so inefficient; none of alternate tribes were slanted to go to war to expel them.) They survived extremely well on a low-calorie diet. At the point when the white men came, be that as it may, carrying their usual eating regimen with them, the Indians got to be fat. Presently more than 90% of them are extremely fat and around the same number experience the ill effects of diabetes. They had developed over numerous eras to live on an inadequate eating regimen. Most likely whatever is left of us are likewise not exactly sufficiently developed to adapt to our advanced eating routine.

3. Exercise is significant. An absence of exercise reasons obesity; and we are showing signs of improvement and better at not getting enough exercise, There are special cases. A mess of individuals are circling, actually, or playing sports, including team activities, at a propelled age. This never used to happen. When I was a child, on the off chance that I saw somebody going through the boulevards of Manhattan, I knew they were running for a transport. Specifically, it is socially satisfactory now for ladies to play sports for the duration of their lives. In this way, there are a minority who are exceptionally dynamic physically. Yet, a more prominent number are less dynamic than individuals used to be. TV normally gets faulted. Before that there was radio. At the point when phones first came in, the vast majority thought the gadget would never get on. On the off chance that they needed to converse with somebody, they said, they could simply stroll over to that individual's home. These days, if individuals truly need to go some place, they drive as opposed to walk, utilize a lift instead of trip stairs and are, when all is said in done, latent as opposed to dynamic.

As time goes on, physical movement affects keeping up appropriate weight that is at any rate as imperative as a legitimate eating regimen.

4. Uncalled for dietary patterns, learned while growing up, are thought to add to exorbitant weight increase through the span of an existence time. The issue arrives is no assention about what constitutes legitimate or inappropriate dietary patterns.

Getting done with eating everything on your plate used to be viewed as great; now it is viewed as terrible. You ought to quit eating when you are no more eager. Try not to eat that last potato on the grounds that it is staying there on your plate. It is regularly prescribed to weight watchers that they get in the propensity for intentionally abandoning some nutrition uneaten on their plates.

5. Another reason given for putting on weight is a lot of TV. The measure of time kids sit in front of the TV has been appeared to associate with weight; the more they watch, the heavier they get. Perhaps the impact is through an absence of exercise. Somebody sitting inactive on a love seat is not outside taking care of business. On the other hand, maybe, the nutrition plugs on TV that are intended to make individuals hungry really do make them hungry.

4. Absence of rest. Individuals who rest less eat more. Possibly they don't have anything better to do. Perhaps there are compound changes that occur in the mind to make up for insufficient rest. There is a voracity focus in the cerebrum, and it is known not influenced by circumstances, including, perhaps, lack of sleep. (The voracity focus in the cerebrum is near the range that controls sex—which ought to say something; yet I don't realize what.)

5. Certain medications. A portion of the antidepressants, for instance, cause weight pick up. Throughout the years I have changed over a couple chronically discouraged, slight ladies into rotund, however merry moderately aged ladies, (despite the fact that they are not sprightly about being pudgy.) There are various different medications that demonstration likewise.

6. The sun-spot cycle. Similarly as I probably am aware, there is no relationship between's sun-spots and weight pick up. I say this here just to keep the peruser's consideration.

7. craziness for meat. Neediness connects with obesity. There are most likely two reasons: there is little access in the inward city to new foods grown from the ground. Handled nourishments are additionally fattening. Furthermore, sound nutritions are more costly, along these lines, in poor groups, a society of eating fricasseed nourishments and other fattening nourishments has grown up.

8. **Certain hormones.** The standard thing "glandular conditions" that are specified frequently by laypeople as a clarification for obesity incorporate low thyroid and high cortisone levels. The impacts they deliver on weight, on the other hand, are moderately minor and conflicting. There are different hormones, be that as it may, emitted in the stomach that are known not ravenousness somehow. Procedures are being produced to control weight utilizing them; however the outcomes so far have been frustrating. The stomach sidestep operations that are utilized as of now to treat horrible obesity are known not these hormones, and it might be in part through that instrument that these operations work.

9. **The microbes that live in the digestive tract.** There are a large number of human cells in the body; however ten times that numerous microorganisms take up habitation in each of us, especially in our digestion systems. These groups of microorganisms fluctuate starting with one individual then onto the next. They help us to process our nutrition, and some are more productive at that assignment than others. In this way, a few individuals, given the same measure of nourishment, ingest a bigger number of calories than others. Along these lines, truly a specific individual can eat practically nothing, not exactly other individuals, and still put on weight.

A study was led in which various individuals ate the same number of calories and exercised to the same degree; yet there was a noticeable distinction in the change of weight every individual experienced! There are just three conceivable reasons why this could happen: for reasons unknown, a few individuals are better at engrossing the calories from their nutrition than others, maybe as a result of those microscopic organisms which help processing. Also, a few individuals are more dynamic when they are resting (not working out) than others. Most likely both of these clarifications are valid. The third reason, a characteristic distinction in digestion system, might bring about a fairly higher body temperature; yet the component of this higher digestion system might in any case boil down to moving indistinctly more than other individuals.

10. **Microorganisms influence weight** secondly: they appear to influence the hormones that the stomach secretes to direct weight. A typical icy infection, adenovirus-36, has been connected to obesity, maybe in light of the fact that it influences the quantity of fat cells in the body.

11. The more noteworthy accessibility of nutrition. In the course of the most recent 50 years, changing horticultural approaches have energized all the more planting of nutrition which then turns out to be more accessible. At the point when nutrition gets to be less expensive, individuals eat more. Sugar might

be particularly essential. A few individuals date the obesity pandemic to the far reaching accessibility of sugar.

12. It appears that understudies pick up a normal of one to three pounds amid their first exposure.

An excessive amount of eating — insufficient development.

At the point when individuals eat an excess of calories in respect to their vitality use — they put on weight.

When they eat less calories than they smolder — they shed pounds.

Today, we're going to take a gander at the primary variables that influence the amount you eat and what number of calories you use.

This won't be a sweeping rundown, however it will give you an essential thought of the diverse components that influence cause a few individuals to convey more muscle to fat quotients than others.

High set point.

Your "set point" is a scope of body fatness that your body tries to keep up over a time of time.1

When you eat a bigger number of calories than you have to keep up this level of muscle to fat quotients, your body rolls out improvements to keep you from putting on weight.

Your body diminishes craving and now and then expands the amount you move to smolder the additional calories.

When you eat less calories than your body needs to keep up this level of muscle to fat quotients, your body rolls out improvements to keep you from getting more fit. It expands your craving levels and diminishes your inspiration to work out.

Both your introductory set point and your body's reaction to changes in calorie admission can be entirely not quite the same as other individuals.

There is a tremendous variety in how individuals react to gorging and under-eating. A few individuals put on weight precisely in extent to the amount they over-eat.2-4 They likewise have a tendency to have a harder time losing this weight.

Others scarcely increase any fat in spite of enormously over-expending calories.5 These individuals additionally tend to effortlessly lose the weight they do pick up.

With the right decisions you can bring down your set point after some time. A standout amongst the best methods for making so as to do this is shrewd nourishment decisions. Tragically, many people don't.

Poor nutrition decisions.

Individuals regularly accept they can eat less and get in shape while eating huge amounts of garbage. They're correct. Be that as it may, they as a rule experience difficulty adhering to this type of eating routine in the long haul.

There's nothing amiss with little indulgences, however you likely won't have the capacity to stick to an eating routine that is based around Ho-Ho's and Coke. You'll get hungry, possibly create supplement inadequacies, and might likewise not expend enough protein to keep up muscle mass.6-9

My custom made fourfold chocolate brownies are powerfully tasty, yet not as filling as meat and vegetables and simple to over-eat. (Like each other nourishment, they're additionally fine in moderation).

Few individuals really eat like that, however regardless they don't settle on awesome nutrition decisions in different ways. Individuals frequently don't eat enough protein, vegetables, natural product, or fiber — and they stay hungry.6,8,10-16 All. The. Time.

These nutritions are more satisfying than the types that are commonplace in most industrialized nations. Eating enough protein is likewise vital to offer you some assistance with maintaining your bulk while dieting.6

Nourishment accessibility additionally decides how much and what you eat. On the off chance that you have loads of delectable fatty nutrition accessible at all times, then it's anything but difficult to indulge garbage food.17,18 For example, on the off chance that you have an enormous stash of Oreos in your storeroom, you're ready to eat a large number of calories with almost no exertion.

Entire nourishments like rice, chicken, or margarine are still simple to plan can at present be a wellspring of overabundance calories. On the off chance that you don't keep a considerable measure of treats in your home, you still most likely have simple access to eateries and fast food.

Another misstep individuals make is that they encompass themselves with an immense astypement of nourishments. This for all intents and purposes dependably makes them eat more than they ought to.

When you have a bigger astypement of nourishment decisions, you eat more without acknowledging it. This is valid for both "solid" and "horrible" foods.

The "quality" of your eating routine (whatever that way to you) doesn't change the amount of weight you lose at a given calorie consumption. It influences the amount you eat, and in this way your capacity to keep up a caloric shortfall after some time.

Affectability to nutrition signals.

Quite a bit of your eating conduct is dictated by nutrition signs — little triggers in your surroundings that instruct you to eat increasingly or less.22-24 Here are some normal nourishment signals that impact the amount you eat:

How quick you eat.

How quick the general population around you eat.

What number of individuals you're eating with.

How occupied you are while eating.

Regardless of whether nourishment is vanishing from your plate.

The size and measurement of the holders you eat out of.

A few individuals eat more because of these nourishment signals than others. They eat increasingly when others eat more, they're all the more effectively diverted while eating, and so forth.

Individuals why should capable notice and comprehend nutrition prompts that offer them some assistance with stopping eating or eat less by and large have a less demanding time maintaing a sound weight and/or getting thinner.

Individuals who are ignorant of nourishment signals or don't react to them, by and large experience more difficulty getting in shape.

Low practice levels.

Janet is an inactive individual who blazes zero calories through formal activity.

Jake is a profoundly prepared continuance competitor who can blaze around 6,000 calories in a solitary workout.

Clearly, Janet and Jake should eat altogether different measures of nourishment. Jake can likewise most likely drop weight quicker than Janet.

These are great illustrations, however the amount you practice has an enormous effect on your capacity to get thinner.

Individuals who don't practice are for the most part at a much higher danger of getting to be overweight, have a harder time shedding pounds, and battle more with keeping up their weight loss.

Individuals who practice routinely have a tendency to lose more weight and keep it off better after some time. You don't need to do much, yet in the event that you need to get in shape, you ought to do some moderate activity all the time.

Low day by day development levels.

Non-exercise action thermogenesis, otherwise known as "Perfect," speaks to the greater part of the calories you smolder from every day developments that don't consider formal exercise.

A few individuals have much more elevated amounts of NEAT than others. They additionally tend to build NEAT while indulging more than other individuals, which offers them some assistance with burning off the additional calories.

Little developments like standing and wriggling can include for the duration of the day, infrequently to right around 1,000 calories.5 People with elevated amounts of NEAT have a much simpler time not putting on weight and getting in shape.

Low levels of restraint.

A few individuals don't have as much restraint, or self discipline, as others and aren't as great at controlling their motivations.

When you consider that you settle on around 200 nutrition related choices for every day,47 this is a conspicuous issue.

The yearning to eat is viewed as the most widely recognized one you encounter, making up around 28% of your day by day urges.48 Most individuals follow up on these desires about portion of the time.

Individuals who are overweight regularly act all the more hastily and don't control their eating and practice practices and additionally incline individuals, and have a harder time losing weight.

They eat the second they get a little appetite longing for.

They eat on the grounds that nourishment is accessible, not on the grounds that they require it.

They eat when they see a fast food eatery, regardless of the possibility that they aren't eager.

When they eat, they frequently forget about their nourishment allow and eat much more than they know they ought to — they have more prominent dietary "disinhibition."

They aren't great at rousing themselves to reliably work out, or practice hard.

They don't stick to eats less in the long haul.

Interestingly, individuals who are told they need determination when they truly don't abandon hard undertakings sooner.

Suppose you have somebody with a lower than ordinary level of discretion. They gorge on a couple events, and perhaps increase some fat. At that point they get furious at themselves and begin to accept they're "powerless willed." This attitude further reductions their self control, and will probably lose control later on.

Their self-uncertainty turns into a type of self-satisfying prescience.

Your capacity to control your practices has an enormous effect on your capacity to keep up a solid weight. It will be less demanding for some, and harder for others, yet it's imperative for everybody.

Low or nonexistent consciousness of calorie, work out, and muscle to fat ratio ratios levels.

The vast majority have no clue the amount they eat. They don't read nutrition names or know what number of calories are in diverse foods. They overlook the amount they ate even minutes after a meal.

Others basically have no clue the amount of aggregate nutrition volume they eat. In the event that you requesting that they recollect the amount they ate the earlier day, they'd presumably think little of their nutrition admission by no less than 25%.

Turning out to be more mindful of your weight, calorie allow, and practice levels can offer you some assistance with losing weight.

Individuals likewise more often than not expect they're practicing significantly more than they truly are, and that they're smoldering more calories amid exercise.

You're unrealistic to roll out an improvement unless you're mindful of motivation to do as such. On the off chance that you don't see (or overlook) the way that you're overweight or not as incline as you'd like, you won't make a move to redress the issue.

This is as valid for super incline individuals as it is for those simply attempting to be sound. Indeed, even muscle heads and competitors frequently forget about their nourishment allow and muscle to fat ratio ratios levels when they're not planning for a particular occasion, and sometimes pick up a considerable measure of fat without taking note. Others experience serious difficulties getting in shape for the same reasons.

Straightforward practices that make you more mindful of your nourishment consumption, exercise levels, and muscle to fat quotient can massively affect your capacity to keep up a sound weight or lose fat.

Keeping a nourishment and/or exercise diary can infrequently twofold the measure of weight individuals lose in free-living conditions. Weighing yourself is likewise essential to offer you some assistance with staying mindful of how you're eating and practice practices impact your muscle to fat ratio levels.

Science essayist Gary Taubes says that the way to weight reduction is no awesome puzzle—just cut the carbs from your eating routine and the weight will fall off. However, haven't we heard that some time recently? Low-carb weight reduction arranges like Atkins and South Beach were extremely popular in the mid 2000's, however they've following gone the method for some trend diets like the Cabbage Soup and Grapefruit diets. In any case, in his new book, Why We Get Fat, Taubes, a smash hit book writer and contributing journalist for Science magazine, contends that nutritions rich in starches are the primary driver of the obesity plague. While some therapeutic specialists assert that cutting carbs can be undesirable, Taubes says that, as per his exploration, everybody's eating regimen ought to basically be low in breads, grains and even organic products. Best Health talked with Taubes about his book and why he battles that carbs make us fat.

Best Health: What' are a percentage of the greatest slip-up individuals make when attempting to shed pounds?

Gary Taubes: Trying to eat less and practice more. The reason individuals are fat in any case isn't on the grounds that they eat a lot of and practice too little. The reason individuals get fat is on account of their fat tissue gets unregulated. Fat-tissue regulation is controlled by the hormone insulin, and we emit insulin in light of the sugars we expend. The reason we get fat is a direct result of sugars; they actually are fattening. So in the event that you would prefer not to be fat, you don't eat them.

The second error is low-fat eating methodologies. These eating regimens are high-carboydrate diets by definition. In the event that you simply attempt to cut fat your of your eating regimen [without slicing calories] then you're going to raise sugars. So now what you're doing to get in shape is doing the definite inverse.

BH: What is it about carbs that makes us fat?

GT: Carbohydrates used to be considered exceptionally fattening. In my book, I cite a line from an article composed by one of the main dietitians in a 1963 issue of the British Journal of Nutrition: "Each lady realizes that starches make them fat." This was the customary way of thinking up until the 1960s.

Fat amassing in the human body is, in every way that really matters, controlled by the hormone insulin. So when you discharge insulin, you store calories as fat and when insulin levels descend, you discharge the fat and copy it. We discharge insulin in light of sugars in the eating regimen. In the event that you look in a therapeutic course reading, it will let you know that insulin makes fat cells fat. It's never been dubious that so as to dispose of fat, you need to lower insulin levels. What's more, in case you're hereditarily inclined to put on weight, eating carbs is the most obvious trigger.

BH: Low-carb weight control plans were entirely famous around 10 years prior, yet they've subsequent to been relinquished. Why have they dropped out of support?

GT: Well, in light of the fact that the foundation loathes them. The issue is that individuals go on the eating routine and not just do their specialists let them know that they're murdering themselves, yet the specialists say it's pretense and every one of your companions believe you're a nourishment fanatic. So there's zero positive input, aside from that you shed pounds and you feel better.

Furthermore, there's additionally a mood to the press, so first [they say] that the Atkins eating regimen is incredible and everybody's doing it, and after that they say it's out of design. Yet, you could go into an eatery and ask the server what number of individuals ask that the bread not be conveyed to their table, and you'll see that many people these days basically don't eat the bread on the table in light of the fact that they believe it's fattening. There's an extensive low-carb group on line—there are huge amounts of low-carb sites.

BH: Why do specialists believe that low-carb weight control plans are deception?

GT: They accept soaked fat reasons coronary illness and it does as such by raising LDL or supposed "terrible" cholesterol. What's more, these low-carb diets have a tendency to be high in immersed fat on the grounds that you're eating eggs, spread and meat. You don't need to eat those nutritions on a low-carb diet—the essential thought is that some carb-rich nourishments are fattening so simply don't eat those nutritions. You could be a veggie lover or a vegetarian and enhance your getting so as to eat regimen free of the desserts, white bread and potatoes.

Another issue is that specialists trust that weight control plans shouldn't be excessively prohibitive on the grounds that then individuals don't keep focused. The similitude I use to question that will be that cigarettes cause lung growth, pretty much as certain carb-rich nourishments make us fat. On the off chance that a specialist has a patient who is smoking cigarettes, he couldn't care less the amount of his satisfaction in life will be decreased on the off chance that he stops smoking. He just says, 'Look, on the off chance that you would prefer not to get lung disease, don't smoke.'

BH: Should everybody take after a low-carb diet?

GT: For somebody why should incline start with, the message is to not run insane with carb-rich nourishments. It isn't so much that pasta is innately terrible and in case you're incline, you can clearly endure it. So in case you're 10 pounds overweight, possibly you should simply quit eating pasta consistently. In any case, somebody who is 100 pounds overweight will be unable to endure any carbs. Then again, another issue is that obesity, coronary illness diabetes, tumor, Alzheimer's—these ailments group together. They used to be known as sicknesses of human advancement, however now they're considered illnesses of the Western eating regimen. The way the medicinal group considers it is that first you begin getting fat and the weight expands your danger of getting these infections. Another approach to consider it is that whatever makes you fat in any case likewise causes these infections. Regardless of the possibility that these carb-rich nutritions don't make you by and by fat, it's feasible that they are the reason for these maladies. Considers have never been done, yet there are great individuals in the disease research field who feel that sugar and refined starches are most likely the reason for malignancy and don't eat them hence.

BH: In the back of your book you depict a low-carb menu arrangement and it is light on products of the soil. In any case, that conflicts with the overwhelming nourishment guidance, which is to increment leafy foods utilization. Could an eating routine low in these nourishments truly be solid?

GT: It all relies on upon what you can by and by endure. Someone who is 100 pounds overweight won't not have the capacity to eat any natural product in light of the fact that the carbs and the fructose in the organic product may trigger an insulin reaction that keeps them fat. Indeed, even green vegetables could be a lot of relying upon that they are so touchy to the carbs. At this moment we have this sweeping proposal that everybody ought to eat as much leafy foods as they need. In any case, the issue is that incline individuals are not the same as fat individuals. Somebody who is extremely overweight needs to make sense of what they can endure.

BH: What are your tips for somebody who needs to begin on a weight reduction diet?

GT: It's not about what you eat, it's about what you don't eat. So the first thing I would do is get the sugar, high-fructose corn syrup and lager out of the eating routine. The second thing is to dispose of the starches and the grains—the bread, pasta, potatoes and rice. Those are truly fattening. What's more, the third thing I would prescribe is to not stress over fat. Fat is really the one supplement that doesn't invigorate insulin emission.

BH: What will you have for supper this evening?

GT: Well, I'm voyaging, so ideally I'll have the capacity to discover an eatery open late where I can get a steak and brocoli or other green vegetable. It's difficult to perceive how that could be more benefits.

Everybody knows a few individuals who can eat dessert, cake, and whatever else they need and still not put on weight. At the other compelling are individuals who appear to put on weight regardless of how little they eat. Why? What permits one individual to stay slight without exertion however requests that another battle to abstain from putting on weight or recovering the pounds he or she has lost beforehand?

On an extremely basic level, your weight relies on upon the quantity of calories you expend, what number of those calories you store, and what number of you consume. Be that as it may, each of these components is affected by a mix of qualities and environment. Both can influence your physiology, (for example, how quick you blaze calories) and in addition your conduct (the types of nourishments you eat, for case). The interaction between every one of these variables starts right now of your origination and proceeds for the duration of your life.

The calorie comparison

The parity of calories put away and blazed relies on upon your hereditary cosmetics, your level of physical movement, and you're resting vitality consumption (the quantity of calories your body smolders while very still). On the off chance that you reliably smolder the greater part of the calories that you expend throughout a day, you will keep up your weight. On the off chance that you devour more vitality (calories) than you use, you will put on weight.

Abundance calories are put away all through your body as fat. Your body stores this fat inside specific fat cells (fat tissue) — either by augmenting fat cells, which are constantly present in the body, or by making a greater amount of them. In the event that you diminish your nourishment allow and expend less calories than you consume, or in the event that you exercise progressively and consume more calories, your body will decrease some of your fat stores. At the point when this happens, fat cells shrink, alongside your waistline.

Genetic effects

To date, more than 400 unique qualities have been ensnared in the advancement of overweight or obesity, albeit just a modest bunch give off an impression of being significant players. Qualities add to obesity from numerous points of view, by influencing voracity, satiety (the feeling of completion), digestion system, nourishment yearnings, muscle to fat ratio ratios appropriation, and the inclination to utilize eating as an approach to adapt to push.

A 2006 report in Science that concentrated more than 900 individuals demonstrated that the individuals who have two duplicates of a particular quality variation (called Insig-2) were 22% more prone to have a BMI higher than 30. Analysts trust the quality variation influences the regulation of another quality included in fat creation. In subsequent investigations of more than 9,000 individuals (counting individuals with Western European lineage, African Americans, and kids), they found that around 10% conveyed two duplicates of the quality variation.

In another 2006 study, distributed in the Proceedings of the National Academy of Sciences, analysts concentrated on the action levels of three unique qualities in fat specimens from individuals who were typical weight, overweight, or hefty. They took fat specimens from around the members' inward organs and under their skin and discovered distinctive levels of movement (known as quality expression) in the diverse examples. In overweight individuals, expanded articulation of two of the qualities corresponded with a propensity to be "apple-molded." These and related studies have offered analysts better some assistance with understanding how and why obesity happens. They might likewise goad the improvement of new weight reduction medications.

The quality of the hereditary impact on weight issue differs a considerable amount from individual to individual. Research proposes that for a few individuals, qualities represent only 25% of the inclination to be overweight, while for others the hereditary impact is as high as 70% to 80%. Having a harsh thought of how vast a part qualities play in your weight might be useful as far as treating your weight issues.

What amount of your weight relies on upon your qualities?

Qualities are likely a critical patron to your obesity in the event that you have most or the majority of the accompanying attributes:

You have been overweight for a lot of your life.

One or both of your folks or a few other blood relatives are essentially overweight. In the event that both of your folks have obesity, your probability of creating obesity is as high as 80%.

You can't get thinner notwithstanding when you expand your physical action and adhere to a low-calorie diet for a long time.

Qualities are presumably a lower giver for you on the off chance that you have most or the majority of the accompanying attributes:

You are emphatically impacted by the accessibility of nourishment.

You are respectably overweight, yet you can get more fit when you take after a sensible eating regimen and exercise program.

You recapture shed pounds amid the Christmas season, in the wake of changing your eating or exercise propensities, or now and again when you encounter mental or social issues.

These circumstances propose that you have a hereditary inclination to be substantial, however it's not all that good that you can't overcome it with some exertion.

At the flip side of the range, you can expect that your hereditary inclination to obesity is unobtrusive if your weight is typical and doesn't increment notwithstanding when you frequently enjoy fatty nourishments and once in a while exercise.

Individuals with just a moderate hereditary inclination to be overweight have a decent risk of eating so as to shed pounds all alone less calories and getting more fiery exercise all the more frequently. These individuals will probably have the capacity to keep up this lower weight.

What are thrifty qualities?

At the point when the prey got away or the products fizzled, how did our progenitors survive? The individuals who could store muscle to fat quotients to live off amid the incline times lived, and the individuals who proved unable, died. This transformative adjustment clarifies why most present day people — around 85% of us — convey purported thrifty qualities, which offer us some assistance with conserving vitality and store fat. Today, obviously, these thrifty qualities are a condemnation as opposed to a gift. Not just is nutrition promptly accessible to us about all day and all night, we don't need to chase or reap it!

Interestingly, individuals with a solid hereditary inclination to obesity will most likely be unable to get in shape with the typical types of eating regimen and exercise treatment. Regardless of the fact that they get more fit, they are more averse to keep up the weight reduction. For individuals with an exceptionally solid hereditary inclination, sheer self discipline is inadequate in neutralizing their propensity to be overweight. Normally, these individuals can keep up weight reduction just under a specialist's direction. They are additionally the destined to require weight reduction drugs or surgery.

The predominance of obesity among grown-ups in the United States has been ascending following the 1970s (see Figure 1). Qualities alone can't in any way, shape or form clarify such a fast ascent. Despite the fact that the hereditary inclination to be overweight changes generally from individual to individual, the ascent in body mass record gives off an impression of being about widespread, cutting over every single demographic gathering. These discoveries underscore the significance of changes in our surroundings that add to the plague of overweight and obesity.

Percent of grown-ups ages 20–74* who were at a solid weight, overweight, or obese†y.

Ecological impacts

Hereditary elements are the powers inside you that offer you some assistance with gaining weight and stay overweight; natural components are the outside strengths that add to these issues. They envelop anything in our surroundings that makes us more prone to eat an excessive amount of or exercise too little. Taken together, specialists imagine that ecological elements are the main thrust for the emotional increment in obesity.

Ecological impacts become possibly the most important factor early, even before you're conceived. Analysts some of the time call these in-utero exposures "fetal programming." Babies of moms who smoked amid pregnancy will probably get to be overweight than those whose moms didn't smoke. The same is valid for infants destined to moms who had diabetes. Specialists trust these conditions might some way or another modify the developing child's digestion system in ways that appear sometime down the road.

After conception, babies who are bosom bolstered for over three months are more averse to have obesity as teenagers contrasted and newborn children who are bosom sustained for under three months.

Youth propensities regularly stay with individuals for whatever is left of their lives. Kids who drink sugary soft drinks and eat fatty, prepared nutritions add to a desire for these items and keep eating them as grown-ups, which has a tendency to advance weight pick up. In like manner, children who stare at the TV and play computer games as opposed to being dynamic might be customizing themselves for a stationary future.

Numerous components of present day life advance weight pick up. So, today's "obesogenic" surroundings urges us to eat progressively and exercise less. What's more, developing confirmation more extensive parts of the way we live —, for example, the amount we rest, our anxiety levels, and other mental variables — can influence weight also.

The nourishment element

By Centers for Disease Control and Prevention (CDC), Americans are eating a larger number of calories all things considered than they did in the 1970s. Somewhere around 1971 and 2000, the normal man added 168 calories to his every day toll, while the normal lady included 335 calories a day. What's driving this pattern? Specialists say it's a mix of expanded accessibility, greater segments, and all the more fatty nourishments.

For all intents and purposes all over the place we go — malls, sports stadiums, motion picture theaters — nourishment is promptly accessible. You can purchase snacks or suppers at roadside rest stops, 24-hour comfort stores, even rec centers and wellbeing clubs. Americans are spending significantly more on nourishments eaten out of the home: In 1970, we burned through 27% of our nutrition spending plan on far from home nourishment; by 2006, that rate had ascended to 46%.

In the 1950s, fast-food eateries offered one bit size. Today, partition sizes have expanded (see Figure 2), a pattern that has overflowed into numerous different nourishments, from treats and popcorn to sandwiches and steaks. A regular serving of French fries from McDonald's contains three times a larger number of calories than when the establishment started. A solitary "super-sized" feast might contain 1,500–2,000 calories — every one of the calories that the vast majority requirement for a whole day. What's more, research demonstrates that individuals will frequently eat what's before them, regardless of the possibility that they're as of now full.

Segment sizes for nourishments usually expended outside the home have expanded throughout the years, and numerous specialists trust this has added to overweight and obesity. Consider an average fast-food feast that comprises of a cheeseburger, French fries, and a pop. In 1955, shoppers were offered one and only divide size. Today they can choose from various bit sizes. The outline above shows how every one of these segments analyze, conforming for size expansion throughout the years.

As anyone might expect, we're additionally eating all the more unhealthy nourishments (particularly salty snacks, soda pops, and pizza), which are considerably more promptly accessible than lower-calorie decisions like plates of mixed greens and entire organic products. Fat isn't as a matter of course the issue; truth be told, research demonstrates that the fat substance of our eating routine has really gone down following the mid 1980s. Yet, some low-fat nourishments are high in calories on the grounds that they contain a lot of sugar to enhance their taste and tastefulness. Truth be told, some low-fat nourishments are really higher in calories than nutritions that are not low fat.

In one year, the normal American grown-up eats 40 pounds of white bread, 41 pounds of potatoes, 30 pounds of cheddar, and 77 pounds of included fats (spread, grease, and cooking oil), and washes it all down with 52 gallons of pop. Genuine, vegetable utilization has ascended by around 12% since 1990 — however 66% of these vegetables take the type of potatoes (counting chips, fries, and pounded potato), chunk of ice lettuce, and other low-supplement decisions.

Taking all things together, the Department of Agriculture reports that nutrition utilization ascended by 8%, or around 140 pounds for each individual every year, amid the 1990s. Our country produces half more nutrition than we require, and the nourishment business burns through $30 billion a year to make sure it doesn't go to squander. It works: In 2001, Americans burned through $110 billion on fast food, up almost twentyfold in only three decades.

The administration's present suggestions for exercise require an hour of moderate to fiery exercise a day. In any case, less than 25% of Americans meet that objective. Then again, a greater number of individuals are practicing than in the late 1980s. By 2004 CDC report, the rate of individuals who say they do no recreation time physical movement, (for example, strolling, playing golf, or cultivating) dropped from a high of 32% in 1989 to 25% in 2002.

Our day by day lives don't offer numerous open doors for movement. Kids don't exercise as much in school, frequently on account of reductions in physical training classes. Numerous individuals drive to work and spend a great part of the day sitting at a work station. Since we work extend periods of time, we experience difficulty finding an ideal opportunity to go to the rec center, play a game, or exercise in different ways.

Rather than strolling to neighborhood shops and toting shopping sacks, we drive to one-stop megastores, where we stop near the passage, wheel our buys in a shopping basket, and commute home. The across the board utilization of vacuum cleaners, dishwashers, leaf blowers, and a large group of different machines requires almost all the physical exertion out of day by day errands.

The issue with TV: Sedentary nibbling

The normal American watches around four hours of TV for every day, a propensity that has been connected to overweight or obesity in various studies. Information from the National Health and

Nutrition Examination Survey, a long haul study observing the soundness of American grown-ups, uncovered that individuals with overweight and obesity invest more energy sitting in front of the TV and playing computer games than individuals of ordinary weight. Sitting in front of the TV over two hours a day likewise raises the danger of overweight in youngsters, even in those as youthful as three years of age.

Part of the issue might be that individuals are sitting in front of the TV as opposed to practicing or doing different exercises that smolder more calories (staring at the TV blazes just marginally a bigger number of calories than resting, and not exactly other stationary interests, for example, sewing or perusing). In any case, nourishment notices likewise might assume a critical part. The normal hour-long TV show highlights around 11 nourishment and drink advertisements, which urge individuals to eat. What's more, studies demonstrate that eating nutrition before the TV empowers individuals to eat more calories, and especially more calories from fat. Actually, a study that restricted the measure of TV children viewed showed this practice offered them some assistance with losing weight — yet not on the grounds that they turned out to be more dynamic when they weren't staring at the TV. The distinction was that the youngsters ate a larger number of snacks when they were sitting in front of the TV than while doing different exercises, even inactive ones.

Push and related issues

Obesity specialists now trust that various diverse parts of American culture might plan to advance weight pick up. Anxiety is an ongoing idea entwining these elements. For instance, nowadays it's typical to work extend periods of time and take shorter or less continuous excursions. In numerous families, both folks work, which makes it harder to discover time for families to shop, plan, and eat solid nourishments together. Round-the-clock TV news implies we hear more incessant reports of youngster snatchings and irregular savage acts. This accomplishes more than expansion stress levels; it additionally makes folks more hesitant to permit kids to ride their bicycles to the recreation center to play. Folks wind up driving children to play dates and organized exercises, which implies less action for the children and more stretch for parents. Time weights — whether for school, work, or family commitments — regularly lead individuals to eat on the run and to give up rest, both of which can add to weight pick up.

A few scientists additionally surmise that the very demonstration of eating sporadically and on the run might add to obesity. Neurological confirmation shows that the cerebrum's natural clock — the pacemaker that controls various other day by day rhythms in our bodies — might likewise direct craving and satiety signals. Preferably, these signs ought to keep our weight unfaltering. They ought to incite us to eat when our muscle to fat ratio ratios falls beneath a specific level or when we require more muscle to fat quotients (amid pregnancy, for instance), and they ought to let us know when we feel satisfied and ought to quit eating. Close associations between the mind's pacemaker and the longing control focus in the hypothalamus propose that yearning and satiety are influenced by fleeting signals. Sporadic eating examples might disturb the viability of these signs in a way that advances obesity.

Chapter 2

Biological mechanism of weight loss

When you read this, the greater part of your patients will have made and broken their New Year's resolutions many times over, and the reason is understood, for the most part on account of its subject: weight reduction. More than 85% pledge to roll out way of life improvements, a considerable lot of these including a guarantee to get in shape. Despite the fact that making a determination has been appeared to be the most intense system for getting in shape, numerous still fizzle. "On the off chance that they could just make a fat pill!" is a cry heard around the New Year from numerous overweight Americans—assessed to be 66% of the present populace.

They are not going to get their pharmacological wish, sadly, for we are no place close making a medicine ensured to dissolve off the pounds. Yet there is each motivation to be hopeful that one may in the long run get to be accessible.

Here I talk about a promising finding: the revelation of a system that makes well evolved creatures impervious to weight increase even notwithstanding a high-fat eating routine. To comprehend this advancement, we will obviously audit some essential science of the hypothalamus and talk about the cooperations of 2 extremely fascinating atoms—a protein called synaptotagmin 4 (Syt4) and maybe the world's most celebrated nonapeptide, oxytocin. Don't hesitate to skip to the area "The information" if the paraventricular hypothalamus and calcium-free presynaptic vesicle combination are working parts of your vocabulary.

The hypothalamus and 2 particles

As you most likely are aware, the hypothalamus is included in the regulation of body weight. Particular accumulations of neurons inside of this multitalented locale are host to a confusing number of metabolic input circles, intervening their consequences for our weight support through the arrival of particular neurotransmitters. These longing particular areas incorporate the paraventricular hypothalamus and the supraoptic core, both of which emit oxytocin.

Oxytocin has gotten a considerable measure of press throughout the years, gathering well known consideration in light of its inclusion in social comprehension. It has been appeared to intervene sentiments of trust in warm blooded animals running from voles to love birds. Be that as it may, oxytocin is additionally included in uterine constrictions for birthing moms (the medication pitocin is a manufactured type of oxytocin) and in the let-down reflex for nursing ones. This renowned particle set off the 1955 Nobel prize in science for Vincent du Vigneaud.

As of late, this flexible polypeptide has been embroiled in obesity, in any event in mouse models. The key finding is that a diminishment in articulation of oxytocin prompts fat creatures. The system includes a criticism projection, for the most part from the paraventricular hypothalamus back to the hindbrain. This is a major ordeal in light of the fact that this neural thruway is included in feast size regulation. Much all the more as of late, the neurons that emit oxytocin have additionally been appeared to express a compound produced using a variation of a quality called FTO. Initially disengaged by a gathering of analysts intrigued by type 2 diabetes mellitus, this variation has been emphatically associated with human obesity. Individuals with 2 duplicates of this allele have very nearly a 2-fold higher rate of obesity than the individuals who don't.

Another particle we have to audit is Syt4. To portray the capacity of this protein in obesity, we have to quickly audit the secretory instruments that prompt neurotransmitter discharge, a procedure in which the synaptotagmin group of particles is profoundly enmeshed.

As you might know, neurotransmitters are put away in oil lined vesicles, restricted to 2 places in presynaptic neurons. Some are in the alleged dynamic zones, near the cell film, where discharge will in the long run happen. Numerous are put away promptly behind these zones, held set up by a protein framework whose parts are by and large called vesicle-related layer proteins.

Neurotransmitters discharge happens when the vesicles in the dynamic zone wire to the presynaptic film and dump their substance into the neurotransmitter. This combination, activated by an inundation of calcium, is interceded by means of a gathering of proteins by and large called the combination complex. A critical individual from this complex is synaptotagmin, whose occupation is to sense calcium and empower the last few stages of neurotransmitter discharge. Without synaptotagmin, there would be no neurotransmitter release.

Syt4 is one individual from a group of synaptotagmin proteins, however it is the odd one out of the tribe. Syt4 can-not sense calcium and, thus, down-controls synaptic arrival of neurotransmitters. This inhibitory capacity will turn out to be an imperative segment in our obesity story (more on that in a moment).

To comprehend the obesity information, we have to survey the particles as well as how they were utilized as a part of the lab. The primary needs to do with an old and settled hereditary building convention known as "thump out" innovation. Without getting impeded in the subtle elements, it is conceivable to make research center creatures (mice) that are impeccably typical all around aside from one: a particular quality has been thumped out of their chromosomal supplement. Expecting the creatures can get by without the quality, the DNA's capacity might be surmised just by looking at any irregularity the creature presents. It is conceivable to make creatures with either one or both qualities missing. In our story, both duplicates of Syt4 have been thumped out, making a creature .

The second piece of innovation includes another survey of your essential atomic science coursework. You review that most qualities have an on/off switch. This switch, only a particular patch of DNA (normally at the leader of the quality) is known as a promoter. On the off chance that you need to express oxytocin, you should turn on the oxytocin promoter, and in the event that you need to express Syt4, you should turn on Syt4s. In the event that you need to turn on Syt4 utilizing signals that ordinarily actuate oxyto-cin expression, you should do some swapping. Essentially sewing the promoter of oxytocin onto the basic quality of Syt4, then bringing this altered quality into whatever phone that intrigues you, will do the trap. The insertion is regularly done by stacking up the mixture develop onto an infection, then permitting the infection to contaminate the cell. The signs that nor-mally drive oxytocin expression might likewise drive Syt4. (See the Figure for further subtle elements.)

In light of these foundation remarks, we are prepared to talk about the discoveries. There are 5 perceptions that make up the majority of the work.1

Perception 1: first intimations. This story begins on a cooperative insight: analysts saw that particular hypothalamic neurons were packed with Syt4 proteins in wild-type creatures, and they had some really world class uncommon organization. Syt4 was colocalized solely with neurons that express oxytocin. This expression profile was so particular (eg, Syt4 was not communicated in neighboring neurons communicating oxytocin-related particles, for example, vasopressin) and the part of oxytocin in weight increase was so settled that it was enticing to examine the part of Syt4 in obesity. Luckily for our story, the specialists respected the allurement.

Perception 2: utilitarian pieces of information section 1. Yet, does this affiliation mean anything practically? The least complex test in obesity examination is to sustain mice a high-fat eating regimen, then see what happens to their brains. That is precisely what the analysts did. They searched for changes in Syt4 expression designs in the vicinity of such caloric presentation in those oxytocin-hypothalamic cells—and hit pay soil. Syt4 was undoubtedly hoisted in the mouse hypothalamus with the presentation of the improved nutrition.

Perception 3: utilitarian intimations section 2. Imagine a scenario where the mice did not have Syt4. Would that make them fat-safe? The scientists next made syt4−/syt4−knockout creatures. These creatures were then encouraged the high-fat eating regimen that makes most mice large. The analysts hit pay soil once more, and with a negative result. These creatures did not get to be stout when bolstered the high-fat eating routine. They were, truth be told, totally ensured! In fact, it created the impression that Syt4 assumed an imperative part in the capacity of advanced nutrition to make creatures fat.

Perception 4: part of oxytocin section 1. Shouldn't something be said about that bothersome oxytocin? Utilizing the promoter-swap innovation, the analysts made a Syt4 auxiliary quality with an oxytocin promoter. This had the impact of rendering the quality touchy to oxytocin signals, over-communicating Syt4. The specialists then utilized an infection to convey the develop to oxytocin neurons in the knockout creatures and unengineered controls. Notwithstanding the hereditary foundation, over-articulation of Syt4 prompted body weight pick up. The scientists could turn around the defensive impacts of the syt4–/syt4–animals. Truth be told, they could kill the impact on and like a light.

Perception 5: part of oxytocin section 2. The above analyses should be possible as a result of another perception in regards to oxytocin: it had been beforehand seen that the Syt4 knockout mice had hoisted levels of oxytocin contrasted and controls. Truth be told, when the analysts gave these knockout mice a high-fat eating regimen, the serum levels of oxytocin were nearly tripled contrasted and controls.

Was the "ordinary" employment of Syt4 to avoid oxytocin discharge? Given its regular (albeit uncommon) inhibitory part, that would bode well. Through another complex arrangement of investigations, that is precisely what the analysts found. Syt4's normal everyday employment might be to avoid oxytocin discharge in the hypothalamus. Maybe that is one motivation behind why the 2 atoms are colocalized. To demonstrate this in a most exquisite design, the scientists gave the knockout creatures a medication that can obstruct the activity of oxytocin (a receptor opponent). To the analysts' pleasure, the defensive impact vanished. These knockout creatures put on weight when bolstered a high-fat eating regimen.

The finding is very clear: Syt4 is significantly included in the systems that control high-fat–mediated obesity.

The component underlining weight reduction instigated by weight reduction surgery can be clarified by examining the adjustments in body pose, and changes in strolling walk that is actuated by obesity surgery.

1) Obesity surgery leaves an injury in the stomach divider and an injury in the stomach.

2) The stomach divider injury mends in a matter of days, however the stomach wound takes any longer and now and again, it neglects to recuperate by any stretch of the imagination.

3) Even when the stomach wound is mended, there are still staples or a band, contingent upon what type of surgery is performed

The stomach divider injury and the stomach wound, and later the staples or other surgical gadgets that is left in the stomach such as lap band and so on., strengths patients to receive a superior body stance in a sitting position, else they will encounter uneasiness or torment in the midriff territory.

Slumped or a to a great degree slumped stance in a sitting position diminishes the measure of the stomach cavity and in the meantime, it modifies the state of the stomach cavity. The injury in the stomach pit and later the surgical gadgets, similar to staples, lap band, and so on.; make the belly more touchy to changes fit as a fiddle and size of the stomach depression.

Due to the injuries, the patient is compelled to keep up an ideal size of the stomach hole; generally the injury will be packed. At the point when the stomach wound is compacted, the patient encounters expanded strain or torment in the guts.

The ideal size of the stomach hole is conceivable to accomplish just by keeping up a decent body stance.

The ideal size and state of the stomach hole is conceivable to accomplish just by an ideal upward lifting movement of the abs.

The stomach divider injury and the stomach wound, and later the staples or other surgical gadgets that is left in the stomach such as lap band and so on invigorate the upward lifting movement of the abs.

an) In many cases, the patient doesn't accomplish a perfect right body stance, however it is compelled to keep up a vastly improved body stance than before obesity surgery.

b) Improving the body pose absolutely influences the size and state of the stomach cavity.

The heaviness of the abdominal area (the part of the body over the mid-region) gives mechanical incitement on the guts just for the situation when it isn't upheld by the abs. At the point when the muscular strength bolster the abdominal area weight, the abdominal area weight doesn't discourage the waistline and mid-region, and that has the result that it doesn't affect mechanical incitements on the guts.

The nonattendance of mechanical incitements is the component that causes weight reduction (relapse of the bone, muscle and fat mass).

A Contributing element for weight reduction after weight reduction surgery is a diminished quality of ground effect strengths. [Any genuine damage, whether it is brought on by a mishap or by surgery, compels an adjustment in the strolling gait].

The stomach divider injury, the stomach wound, and later the staple or other surgical gadgets that are left in the stomach such as lap band and so forth., drives patients to take more care of how he exchanges his body weight from one leg to the next.

Before obesity surgery, the patient could walk while keeping up a pretty much unequal strolling and running step (pretty much ungainly stride).

After obesity surgery, strolling with an unequal stride will create uneasiness or torment in the stomach area. The injury in the belly, later the staples or lap band, compels the patient to stroll in a manner that he exchanges the body weight from one leg to the next in a more adjusted manner then before weight reduction surgery.

The injury in the stomach compels the patient to perform a more productive headway than what was the situation before obesity surgery, and after the injury recuperates the staples, lap band and so on that is left in the stomach or in the stomach hole, drives the patient to perform a more proficient velocity than what was the situation before obesity surgery.

The step change causes an enhanced proficiency of strolling (productivity of motion).

The enhanced productivity of headway reasons decreased quality of the ground sway strengths.

The lessened quality of effect powers causes diminished quality of the mechanical incitements.

Diminished quality and/or length of time of mechanical incitements beneath the level essential for keeping up the current body mass will bring about the loss of muscle, bone and fat mass.

To completely comprehend the instrument underlining weight reduction prompted by Weight Loss Surgeries, it is important to know a tad bit about mechanical incitement.

In weightlessness, the human body is presented to just about a complete nonappearance of mechanical incitement, in light of the fact that in weightlessness the body does not have weight and there is no ground sway power.

On Earth, the human body is presented to four types of mechanical incitements.

1. Mechanical incitements – type 1 are created by the heaviness of the body.

The human body is presented to mechanical incitement type 1, while resting, sitting and for the season of performing headway, such as strolling, running, bouncing, and so on.

2. Mechanical incitement – type 2 are created by a ground sway drive that seems every time when we exchange the heaviness of the body from one leg to the next.

To get the thought of what the ground sway power is, it is sufficient to hit the ground with the base of the feet and you will feel how the effect power transmits from the base of the feet all through whatever remains of the body.

By watching overweight or corpulent individuals when they walk or run, we can see that by exchanging the body weight from one leg to the next they, to some degree, tumble from one leg to the next like they are venturing harder on the ground with their feet, and that has the outcome of delivering more grounded ground sway strengths.

a) When fighters are walking, they hit the ground with their feet. Yet, there are immense contrasts between a warrior's walk and a lopsided stride. While walking, the officers utilize their bones and muscles to strike the ground and in the meantime, to move themself starting with one place then onto the next by exchanging their body weight from one leg to the next.

b) A rearranged clarification of what happens while strolling with an unequal stride would be; the heaviness of the body strikes the ground by tumbling from one leg to the next.

3. Mechanical incitements – type 3 is delivered by the wiggling of fat tissues.

Generally, mechanical incitements – type 3 is a side result of the effect power consolidated with development of the body parts. Among amazingly fat individuals, it is discernible that notwithstanding when they are in a resting position, that by every development of any parts of the body, such as moving the arm, it creates a shaking of the fat tissues.

By essentially watching corpulent individuals when they are strolling, it is outwardly observable how their fat tissues are shaking with every stride they make.

4. Mechanical incitements – type 4 are impelled by the pressure of muscles and fat tissues.

For instance; rolling the pelvis completely in reverse will lessen the vertical size of the waistline.

Chapter 3

The food and nutrition for weight loss

Here are the 20 most weight reduction well disposed nutritions on earth, that are bolstered by science.

1. Full Eggs

Once dreaded for being high in cholesterol, entire eggs have been making a rebound.

New studies demonstrate that they don't unfavorably influence blood cholesterol and don't bring about heart assaults (1, 2).

Furthermore... they are among the best nutritions you can eat in the event that you have to get thinner.

They're high in protein, sound fats, and can make you feel full with a low measure of calories.

One investigation of 30 overweight ladies demonstrated that having eggs for breakfast, rather than bagels, expanded satiety and made them eat less for the following 36 hours (3).

An additional 8 week study found that eggs for breakfast expanded weight reduction on a calorie confined eating regimen contrasted with bagels (4).

Eggs are likewise extraordinarily supplement thick and can offer you some assistance with getting every one of the supplements you require on a calorie confined eating regimen. All the supplements are found in the yolks.

2. Verdant Greens

Kale

Verdant greens incorporate kale, spinach, collards, swiss chards and a couple of others.

They have a few properties that make them ideal for a weight reduction diet.

They are low in both calories and sugars, however stacked with fiber.

Eating verdant greens is an awesome approach to build the volume of your dinners, without expanding the calories. Various studies demonstrate that dinners and diets with a low vitality thickness make individuals eat less calories generally speaking (5).

Verdant greens are additionally fantastically nutritious and high in a wide range of vitamins, minerals and cancer prevention agents. This incorporates calcium, which has been appeared to help fat smoldering in a few studies (6).

3. Salmon

Slick fish like salmon is fantastically sound.

It is additionally extremely fulfilling, keeping you full for a long time with generally couple of calories.

Young lady with Salmon

Salmon is stacked with fantastic protein, sound fats furthermore contains a wide range of vital supplements.

Fish, and fish by and large, supplies a lot of iodine.

This supplement is vital for appropriate capacity of the thyroid, which is critical to keep the digestion system running ideally .

Concentrates on demonstrate that countless on the planet aren't getting all the iodine they require .

Salmon is additionally stacked with Omega-3 fatty acids, which have been appeared to decrease aggravation, which is known not a noteworthy part in obesity and metabolic illness .

Mackerel, trout, sardines, herring and different types of slick fish are additionally superb.

4. Cruciferous Vegetables

Broccoli

Cruciferous vegetables incorporate broccoli, cauliflower, cabbage and brussels grows.

Like different vegetables, they are high in fiber and have a tendency to be unbelievably satisfying.

Additionally... these types of veggies likewise have a tendency to contain better than average measures of protein.

They're not as high in protein as creature nourishments or vegetables, yet they're high contrasted with most vegetables.

A mix of protein, fiber and low vitality thickness makes cruciferous vegetables the ideal nourishments to incorporate into your suppers in the event that you have to get in shape.

They are additionally very nutritious, and contain disease battling substances (11).

5. Incline Beef and Chicken Breast

Lady Eating Meat

Meat has been unreasonably slandered.

It has been reprimanded for a wide range of wellbeing issues, in spite of no great confirmation to back it up.

Albeit handled meat is unfortunate, concentrates on demonstrate that natural red meat does NOT raise the danger of coronary illness or diabetes (12, 13).

By huge survey examines, red meat has just an extremely powerless relationship with tumor in men, and no connection at all in ladies (14, 15).

Actually… meat is a weight reduction neighborly nourishment, on the grounds that it's high in protein.

Protein is the most satisfying supplement, by a wide margin, and eating a high protein eating regimen can make you wreck to 80 to 100 more calories for every day (16, 17, 18).

Ponders have demonstrated that expanding your protein admission to 25-30% of calories can cut yearnings by 60%, lessen wish for late-night nibbling significantly, and cause weight reduction of right around a pound for each week… just by adding protein to the eating routine (19, 20).

In case you're on a low-carb diet, then don't hesitate to eat fatty meats. In any case, in case you're on a moderate-to high starch diet, then picking incline meats might be more proper.

6. Bubbled Potatoes

Potatoes

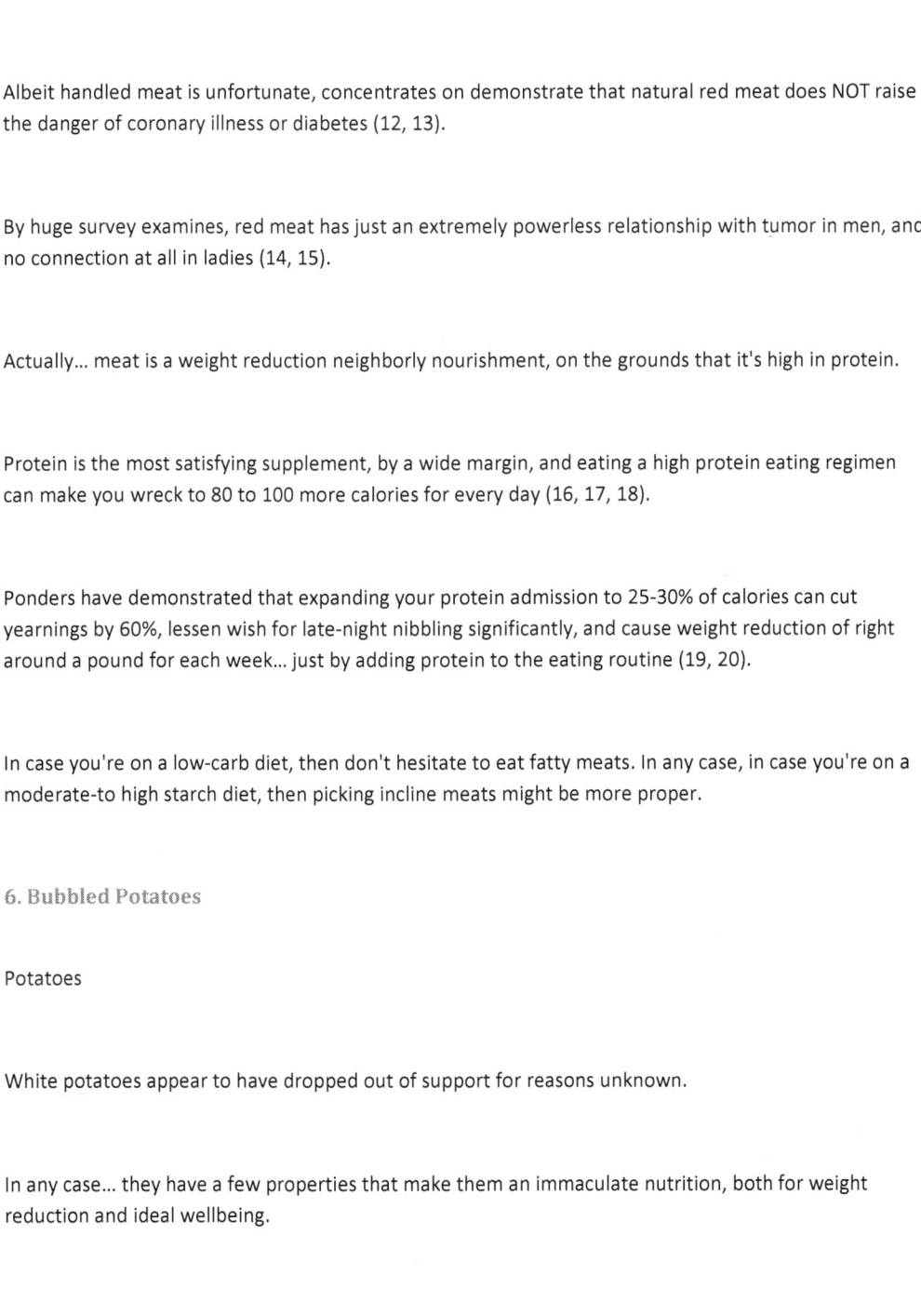

White potatoes appear to have dropped out of support for reasons unknown.

In any case… they have a few properties that make them an immaculate nutrition, both for weight reduction and ideal wellbeing.

They contain an inconceivably astypeed scope of supplements, a tiny bit of practically all that we require.

There have even been records of individuals living on only potatoes alone for broadened timeframes.

They are especially high in potassium, a supplement that a great many people don't get enough of and assumes an imperative part in circulatory strain control.

On a scale called the Satiety Index, that measures how satisfying distinctive nutritions are, white, bubbled potatoes scored the most noteworthy of the considerable number of nourishments tried (21).

This means by eating white, bubbled potatoes, you will actually feel full and eat less of different nourishments.

On the off chance that you heat up the potatoes, then permit them to cool for some time, then they will frame a lot of safe starch, a fiber-like substance that has been appeared to have a wide range of medical advantages... including weight reduction (22).

Sweet potatoes, turnips and other root vegetables are likewise superb.

7. Fish

Fish

Fish is another low-calorie, high protein nutrition.

It is incline fish... so there isn't much fat in it.

Fish is mainstream among muscle heads and wellness models who are on a cut, in light of the fact that it's an awesome approach to keep protein high, with aggregate calories and fat low.

In case you're attempting to underline protein admission, then make a point to pick fish canned in water, yet not oil.

8. Beans and Legumes

Kidney Beans

A few beans and vegetables can be gainful for weight reduction.

This incorporates lentils, dark beans, kidney beans and a few others.

These nourishments have a tendency to be high in protein and fiber, which are two supplements that have been appeared to prompt satiety.

They additionally have a tendency to contain some safe starch.

The primary issue is that many individuals have issue enduring vegetables. Thus, it is vital to set them up appropriately.

9. Soups

A Bowl of Vegetable Soup

As specified above, suppers and diets with a low vitality thickness tend to make individuals eat less calories.

Most nutritions with a low vitality thickness are those that contain loads of water, for example, vegetables and natural products.

Be that as it may, you can likewise simply add water to your nourishment... by making a soup.

A few studies have demonstrated that eating precisely the same, with the exception of made in a soup rather than as strong nutrition, makes individuals feel more satisfied and eat fundamentally less calories.

10. Curds

Curds

Dairy items have a tendency to be high in protein.

One of the best ones is curds... calorie for calorie, it is for the most part only protein with next to no sugar and fat.

Eating a lot of curds is an extraordinary approach to support your protein admission. It is additionally extremely satisfying, making you feel full with a moderately low measure of calories.

Dairy items are likewise high in calcium, which has been appeared to help in the fat blazing procedure .

11. Avocados

Avocados are a novel type of organic product.

Lady Holding a Green Avocado

While most natural product is high in carbs, avocados are stacked with solid fats.

They are especially high in monounsaturated oleic corrosive, the same kind of fat found in olive oil.

Regardless of being for the most part fat, they additionally contain a great deal of water, so they aren't as vitality thick as you might think.

Avocados are immaculate as augmentations to plate of mixed greens, in light of the fact that studies demonstrate that the fats in them can expand the supplement uptake from the vegetables 2.6 to 15-fold.

They likewise contain numerous essential supplements, including fiber and potassium.

12. Apple Cider Vinegar

Decanter With Apple Cider Vinegar

Apple juice vinegar is extraordinarily famous in the common wellbeing group.

It is prevalent for use in sauces, similar to dressings or vinaigrettes. A few individuals even weaken it in water and drink it.

A few studies in people recommend that vinegar can be helpful for individuals why should attempting get thinner.

Taking vinegar in the meantime as a high-carb dinner can build sentiments of totality and make individuals eat 200-275 less calories for whatever remains of the day (26, 27).

One study in corpulent people additionally demonstrated that 15 or 30 mL of vinegar for every day for 12 weeks brought about weight reduction of 2.6-3.7 pounds, or 1.2-1.7 kilograms (28).

Vinegar has additionally been appeared to lessen glucose spikes after suppers, which might prompt a wide range of helpful consequences for wellbeing in the long haul (29, 30).

13. Nuts

Almonds

In spite of being high in fat, nuts are not inalienably fattening.

They're a fantastic nibble, containing adjusted measures of protein, fiber and solid fats.

Thinks about have demonstrated that eating nuts can enhance metabolic wellbeing and even cause weight reduction (31, 32).

Populace considers have additionally demonstrated that individuals who eat nuts have a tendency to be more advantageous, and leaner, than the general population who don't (33).

Simply make a point not to go over the edge, as they are still really high in calories. On the off chance that you tend to orgy and eat gigantic measures of nuts, then it might be best to keep away from them.

14. Some Whole Grains

These sweet, succulent summer berries are heavenly both new and dried in trail blend or in a plate of mixed greens, says Lisa Dorfman, an enlisted dietitian and creator of The Reunion Diet. "At only 43 calories for each 3.5 oz serving, they contain 61 percent of the RDA for vitamin C, and they're likewise crammed with potassium, fiber, and resveratrol, a phytonutrient appeared to ensure the heart."

Cilantro

"Cilantro has various medical advantages and is pressed with supplements, for example, fiber, iron, thiamine, zinc, folate, phosphorous, folate, vitamin K, and then some," says Ellis. Also, it has an extraordinary fragrance and flavor that shouts summer! Cilantro might expand the creation of digestive acids, which can invigorate the gut to move waste out. A sound digestive tract is key for weight reduction, says Ellis.

"This sweet tropical organic product is the ideal element for summer smoothies and juices," says Beth Aldrich, an affirmed all encompassing wellbeing and nourishment instructor, and writer of the book Real Moms Love to Eat. "It contains the proteolytic catalyst bromelain, which helps in the processing of protein and blood clump arrangement. As a mitigating super nutrition, pineapple can lessen swelling and thus, you'll have a compliment gut."

Jicama

Otherwise called yam or yambean, this Mexican turnip is an extraordinary wellspring of fiber, says Dr. Jaime Schehr, an enrolled dietitian in New York City. "This plant is awesome for weight reduction because of its high fiber to sugar proportion (an incredible 32g of fiber for each medium jimaca—that is just about a whole day's worth). They are likewise a decent wellspring of potassium, a fundamental mineral in keeping up water equalization in our body."

Ceviche

Ceviche is a great incline protein source found on numerous Mexican menus all through the mid year months, and it's anything but difficult to make at home, says Sharon Richter, an enrolled dietitian in

New York City. Contingent upon what type of fish is utilized, ceviche can extend between 120-175 calories for every serving. (Also, word has it that Lady Gaga energizes up on ceviche while on visit).

Astringent Melon

This astringent and marginally sweet melon is regularly found in Asian advertises and enhances absorption and lower glucose. "Holding glucose under control is imperative in the event that you need to get more fit," says Nicole Kuhl, a clinical nutritionist and Director of Nutrition at Lifespan Medicine. "An excessive amount of sugar in the circulation system sends a sign to the pancreas to discharge the fat putting away hormone insulin. By holding your glucose under control, you will lessen the probability of putting away calories as fat." Can't stomach the sharpness? Have a go at absorbing it chilled saltwater for a couple of hours before eating (crude or cooked).

"Mangoes are an extraordinary approach to fulfill a sweet tooth and to avert different desires," says Rania Batayneh, MPH, a nutritionist and proprietor of Essential Nutrition for You. Mangoes are high in fiber, magnesium, cancer prevention agents, and iron (making them an awesome nibble for ladies who might have iron insufficiency or pallor), says Batayneh. "What's more, in light of the fact that mangoes help in processing, you need to concentrate on eating the natural product versus simply drinking the juice."

Purple Carrots

You know carrots are beneficial for you, yet did you realize that purple carrots are shockingly better? "Purple carrots contain the greater part of the phytochemicals found in orange carrots, and they likewise contain anthocyanins, which are intense cell reinforcements," says Dr. Robert Rey, a Beverly Hills plastic specialist, unscripted television star of Dr. 90210, and creator of Body by Rey.This sweet, crunchy nibble is stacked with effective hostile to maturing properties and ensures against harm brought about by oxidation (free radicals).

This fiber-and potassium-rich organic product makes the ideal summer nibble. At around 170 calories for 8 oz, you can eat only them, in servings of mixed greens, in grains, or wrapped in prosciutto (simply don't snatch a Fig Newton—you'll get more nutrition and less fat from the real natural product).

Wild Alaskan Salmon

"Research distributed in the Journal of Nutrition in 2006 found that the kind of DHA omega-3 oil found in salmon might have an 'against obesity impact' by keeping an expansion in fat cells, bringing about death of pre-fat cells, and advancing the breakdown of fat in the body," says Maleeff. Not certain how to set it up? Attempt any (or all) of these five wonderful salmon formulas.

Peaches

"Stuffed with essential supplements including vitamins An and C, potassium, and iron, one medium peach (just 38 calories) gives about 2 grams of fiber," says Lauren O'Connor, an enrolled dietitian in Los Angeles, California. "A peach gives delicate purgative and diuretic properties; and on account of it's beta carotene, it likewise offers your skin some assistance with staying new and brilliant." (They additionally make the ideal solidified treat! Attempt this formula for pomegranate-peach-sicles).

Sweet Peppers

Peppers are an extraordinary weight reduction nutrition since all astypements contain capsaicin, a characteristic digestion system supporter, says Lisa C. Cohn, an enlisted dietitian and proprietor of Park Avenue Nutrition in New York. Include them into salsa or eat them crisp, broiled, or stuffed to procure their better-body advantages.

Plums

Brimming with supplements and phytochemicals, plums are light in calories however substantial on flavor. What's more, they additionally make an awesome sweet! Enjoy without demolishing your eating routine with this formula for Alsatian plum cakes.

Delicate Shell Crab

Crab is a light, incline wellspring of protein, says Richter. Simply make certain to avoid breaded, floured, or singed astypements to keep it low fat and swimming outfit inviting!

Nectarines

These sweet (and fluff free), low-cal organic products are loaded with flavonoids, lycopene, and lutein, which anticipate ailment and keep your eyes sound. (We simply adore this nectarine and hazelnut plate of mixed greens!)

Watermelon

"Watermelon is my most loved late spring pound-shedding nourishment," says Jennifer Cassetta, a Clinical Nutritionist and proprietor of Health and the City in New York City. Watermelon is 92 percent water—it tops you off, is low in calories yet still contains incredible measures of supplements and growth battling cancer prevention agents like Vitamin C and lycopene.

Corn

"Corn is a starch that opposes increasing so as to process and thusly can help weight reduction safety, controlling glucose levels, and expanding satiety," says Marissa Vicario, a confirmed all encompassing wellbeing mentor and author of Marissa's Well-Being and Health.

Garden Peas

"Peas have higher protein and iron levels than most vegetables, so they can be a decent wellspring of supplements—and a distinct option for non-creature nutritions which have a tendency to be higher in soaked fat," clarifies Vicario.

Green Beans

This late spring veggie staple is an incredible low cal and fat free wellspring of fiber and iron, says Vicario. Not a fanatic of green beans? Shroud them in this generous and sound bean serving of mixed greens (an extraordinary lighter different option for potato plate of mixed greens for picnics).

Turnips

Did you know turnips could help you shed midsection fat? Their high vitamin C and phytochemical levels detoxify your body—and an excess of poisons in the body can prompt fat aggregation around your waist, says Maleeff. At just 34 calories and 8 grams of sugars for each container (versus a potato's 113 calories and 26 grams of starches), have a go at making crushed turnips rather than pureed potatoes for a supplement thick, low-calorie elective, recommends Maleeff.

Grapes

Rich in vitamin C and phytochemicals with cancer prevention agent and hostile to inflammatory properties, grapes might likewise secure against Type 2 diabetes, says Kara Ellis, an enlisted dietitian in New York City. "Grapes likewise have a high water content, making them an invigorating summer nibble that offers you some assistance with feeling full and fulfilled (some new grapes contain just 100 calories)."

Sweet Potatoes

"Sweet potatoes are an incredible wellspring of dietary fiber, which diminishes glucose and insulin spikes, at last decreasing tummy fat," clarifies Shana Maleeff a dietitian and wellness proficient in New York City. Maleeff proposes substituting a sweet potato for potato plate of mixed greens, potato chips, or pureed potatoes at BBQs to spare several calories. (We additionally cherish this formula for squashed cooked sweet potatoes).

Salsa

"Salsa is low in calories and tastes extraordinary on a wide range of solid nourishments (vegetables, servings of mixed greens, poultry, and fish). It has cancer prevention agents, for example, lycopene, which help in cell wellbeing. Use salsa set up of other unhealthy plunges, for example, hummus, onion plunges, and cheddar plunges and you're ensured to cut calories," says Ellis. Make your own at home with this simple formula for hot corn salsa.

"For around 150 cal per 3.5 oz serving, cold singe joins the positions of heart-solid nourishments as a rich wellspring of omega-3 fatty acids. Picking fish over red meat lessens soaked fats in the eating routine and might bring down danger of coronary illness and growths," says O'Connor. High in two types of solid, temperament improving omega-3's (EPA and DHA) this high-protein, low-calorie fish makes an extraordinary fundamental course.

Catfish

This additional incline fish is loaded with vitamin B12, phosphorous, and selenium, and most ranch raised catfish are low in mercury. Skirt the profound fryer to keep it incline, and have a go at flame broiling up some catfish with this yummy marinade.

Rainbow Trout

At just 130 calories for a 3 oz bit, this mellow fish is low in fat and stuffed with protein. It's an extraordinary substitute for high-fat meats such as cheeseburgers, frankfurters, ribs, and sausage, says Maleeff. Toss it on the barbecue for a flavorful, low-fat summer BBQ principle dish.

Burgers

This mid year most loved doesn't need to wreck your waistline! "Utilizing incline ground hamburger (95 percent incline versus 80 percent) for your ground sirloin sandwiches will spare you 170 calories and 19 grams of fat for a 6-ounce burger," says Maleeff. Trench the bun, swap ketchup for tomatoes, and wrap it up in lettuce for a burger that is loaded with flavor, not exhaust calories. Attempt some of these delectable, thinned down burger formulas today evening time.

Blackberries

"A measure of blackberries has just 62 calories and is stuffed with fiber and phytochemicals, including capable flavonoids and anthocyanins, which speed stool and poisons through your digestive framework," says Maleeff. Their high water and fiber content, in addition to sweet taste, make them the ideal invigorating summer weight reduction nutrition. (These blackberry yogurt cheesecake parfaits are ideal for sweet!)

Lima Beans
Lima beans are extraordinary veggie lover wellsprings of protein (one glass offers 15 grams, or the same as 2 ounces of meat). The without fat beans are likewise stuffed with solvent fiber and iron to give long haul vitality and fulfillment.

Walnuts
Brimming with fiber and heart-solid fats (counting omega-3's, which have appeared to have metabolic-boosting advantages), walnuts are awesome to smash on rather than "terrible" fat-filled and salted potato chips, says Maleeff. Simply watch your bit size since nuts are high in calories. (We prescribe preparing a modest bunch into a plate of mixed greens to include crunch and season).

Portabello Mushrooms
A "substantial" vegan distinct option for burgers, barbecued portabella mushrooms are high in fiber and low in calories, says Mindy Hahn, an authorized dietitian situated in Chicago. (They are likewise astonishing stuffed! We cherish this low-fat formula for stuffed portabellas.)

Melon
Actually sweet and high in water content, melon is an extraordinary summer distinct option for fatty and high-fat pastries like frozen yogurt and cakes, says Maleeff. "Appreciate this wonderful melon for treat, and watch the pounds tumble off!"

Crawfish
At just 70 calories and 15 grams of protein for every 3-ounce serving, these minimal lobster-like animals are low calorie and lower in cholesterol than shrimp, says Richter.

Sardines
While they may not be the most appealing thing on the rundown, on the off chance that you can stomach them, pop open a container of sardines this late spring! Sardines are brimming with fat-battling intensifies that balance out glucose. They're rich wellsprings of CO catalyst Q10, vitamin B12, selenium,

omega-3 oils, calcium, phosphorus, and vitamin D. Also, sardines are satisfying and stuffed with protein, says Richter.

Gazpacho

Made of for the most part vegetables and flavors, gazpacho is loaded with water, fiber, and cell reinforcements, making it a low-calorie, filling choice that can supplant more caloric and fattening nourishments in your eating regimen, says Maleeff. Besides, a late Penn State study found that eating a low-calorie soup (like Gazpacho) before a dinner could offer you some assistance with consuming 20 percent less calories at mealtimes.

Bananas

"Bananas contain a little measure of fiber and safe starch, which have gotten late consideration for their potential part in boosting weight reduction," says Ellis. Eating on bananas is simple, advantageous, and low cal. They're additionally an awesome wellspring of potassium, which can be lost in sweat amid intense workouts or on hot summer days. Additionally they make for pleasant beverages, similar to the Jamba Juice Triple Revitalizer with carrot and squeezed orange.

Summer Squash "One serving of summer squash (½ glass) is just 10 calories and contains 15 percent of your every day needs of vitamin C," says Ellis. "Barbecue it, add it to servings of mixed greens, or puree it and add it to heating. Summer squash is a low-calorie, supplement rich nutrition that shouts summer—actually!"

Cabbage

Notwithstanding being nutritious, low-cal and brimming with fiber, cabbage is likewise a top wellspring of sulfur, a mineral our bodies use to create the normal hair-and-nail strengthener keratin, says Rey. To stay thin and appreciate more excellent hair and nails, throw together some vinegar-based coleslaw. Simply avoid rich coleslaw; it can contain an incredible 19 grams of fat for every container!

Arugula

"At a modest 20 calories for each 3 glasses, arugula gives a magnificent wellspring of folate, vitamins An and C, and more than 100 percent of your every day vitamin K needs," says Rey. Not just is it an awesome weight reduction nutrition, arugula can likewise diminish your danger of bone cracks this mid year: A late Framingham Heart study found that individuals who devoured roughly 250 micrograms for every day of vitamin K had a 35-percent lower danger of hip breaks contrasted with the individuals who expended only 50 micrograms for each day, says Rey.

Romaine Lettuce

"One measure of destroyed Romaine lettuce is a minor 10 calories," says Victoria Shanta Retelny, creator of The Essential Guide to Healthy Healing Foods. It's likewise loaded with vitamins and has more fiber than it's other verdant partners, so on the off chance that you are eager, prepare up a serving of mixed greens with a sprinkle of vinegar and oil for a filling, light feast or nibble.

Thyme
"High in flavor, vitamin K, manganese, and iron, thyme is a herb with unpredictable oils, which bolster cells (particularly in the mind) and secure films which can endure when you consume less calories," says Cohn. "Also, thyme is delectable, and keeping your nutrition divine is a key to weight reduction." We concur!

Turkey
"Turkey is an extraordinary wellspring of B vitamins, selenium, and incline protein," says Ellis. Flame broil up a turkey burger (make sure to check for 90-percent incline—or more—on the name) rather than a full-fat ground sirloin sandwich for a lighter, leaner alternative.

Celery
"Albeit accessible year–round, celery is best in the late spring," says Ellis. This super low-calorie nourishment is additionally an astounding wellspring of vitamins K and C, and a decent wellspring of numerous other fundamental supplements, for example, dietary fiber, folate, potassium, and thiamine. "Crunching on celery is one of the most established eating regimen traps in light of the fact that it might diminish general calorie utilization and help in sound absorption."

Lemons and Limes
Both lemons and limes are fantastic wellsprings of Vitamin C, says Ellis, however it's their flavor that guides in weight reduction the most. "We've all been advised to drink loads of water, yet in some cases water's dull taste causes us to swing to different refreshments. Add lemon or lime juice to support your water's flavor and can offer you some assistance with drinking all the more—staying hydrated might stifle hunger, says Ellis.

Wheat

Wheat regularly gets unfavorable criticism with regards to weight reduction, however it can offer fundamental supplements that are useful for health food nuts, says Cohn. The entire grains found in wheat, (for example, bulgur) are incredible wellsprings of vitality, as they are high in B vitamins, minerals, and fiber.

Oats
An awesome vitality source and normally high in solvent fiber (the goopy, thick fiber that advances great absorption), oats are an incredible weight reduction nourishment since such a variety of eating methodologies cause clogging, says Cohn. Eat them as a supporting hot breakfast oat or dry as granola.

Oregano

This delightful, simple to utilize herb is rich in vitamin K, cancer prevention agents, minerals, and omega-3 oils, says Cohn. "Also, the normal fragrant healing of oregano fulfills you an eater—key for long haul achievement."

This incline meat is a decent wellspring of protein and minerals, says Cohn. "3 ounces has 2.5 grams of fat and 143 calories (1/3 the fat of hamburger or pork and 40 percent less calories). Buffalo is generally much lower in hormones and raised on cleaner food."

Yogurt

Yogurt contains normal probiotics, which can diminish tummy bloating, gas and stoppage (frequently hazardous while counting calories). Simply pick Greek astypements, which are higher in protein, lower in included sugar, and velvety, prescribes Cohn.

Prunes

While they needn't bother with a "season," these sweet little treats are an extraordinary weight reduction nourishment. "They're high in great fiber, which keeps you full and fulfilled longer. Along these lines, you won't be enticed to take advantage of those oily potato chips too early after supper. Prunes are likewise high in vitamins and de-bloating potassium (to keep those abs looking fab!)," says Lauren Slayton, a nutritionist in New York City.

Chapter 4

Natural herbs for weight loss
Step by step instructions to Lose Weight Naturally (22 Home and herbal Remedies)

Weight reduction In the Everyday Roots Book I start the part on weight reduction by expressing that I accept there are just two approaches to genuinely oversee weight, through practicing and practicing good eating habits. There just is no enchantment alternate route, keeping in mind this might appear glaringly evident to a few individuals it is disregarded far, far, time after time. Presently you're most likely pondering, if eat less and exercise are the main approaches to get thinner, why did you compose this rundown? Since there are still normal cures and formulas that will offer you some assistance with reaching your definitive objective. In the event that you utilize these notwithstanding eating better and getting some exercise, they can accelerate the procedure. There are various contributing elements to losing/putting on weight, so the beneath cures cover a wide range.

Figure out how to get in shape normally. Extraordinary for any individual who needs to drop two or three pounds or roll out a complete life improvement...

Before you go on you ought to have a basic comprehension of the procedure your body experiences while dropping the pounds. Fat (alongside protein and starches) is put away vitality, plain and straightforward. Calories are the unit that is utilized to gauge the potential vitality in said fats, carbs, and proteins. Your body will change over fat to usable vitality through a progression of substance procedures, and any abundance vitality (calories) that you don't need will be put away. To get in shape, you should use more vitality (or calories) than you take in. When you are utilizing more than you taking as a part of, your body attracts on put away fat to change over it to vitality, which makes the fat cells shrink. It doesn't vanish; it basically changes structure, similar to water to steam. While this is the essential procedure, you likewise need to consider hereditary and natural components. How well the above procedure happens varies from individual to individual.

1. Cinnamon Tea

Glucose directly affects your weight as it influences how hungry and how vivacious you are (whether you have vitality you're significantly more liable to exercise!) If your glucose is adjusted you are more averse to have a disproportionally extensive craving, and your body will be more adept to utilize fat (vitality) instead of putting away it. While banter about its viability delays, more preparatory studies are turning out demonstrating that cinnamon can oversee glucose levels, so why not throw together a fiery cinnamon tea?

You will require...

- 1 teaspoon of ground cinnamon

- 1 cinnamon stick

- 8 ounces of new water

Bearings

Place the cinnamon in a mug and cover with 8 ounces of bubbling water. Steep for 15 minutes before straining. Drinking 1-2 times each day.

Cinnamon Metabolism Tea

2. Green Tea and Ginger

Green tea has long been bantered as a weight reduction help, and more research is expected to affirm or deny how well it functions. While a few studies have turned up nothing, others have distinguished three principle segments in green tea that could oversee weight-caffeine, catechins, and theanine. Caffeine is only a general help to your framework, and speeds up various substantial procedures, including digestion system identified with weight (in fact talking, digestion system alludes to all natural procedures in a living creature expected to manage life.)

Catechins are viewed as hostile to oxidant flavonoids, and are predominant in green tea instead of dark tea because of a distinction in handling (dark tea is matured.) While the instrument is yet to be resolved, in vitro and in vivo concentrates on have demonstrated that catechins can bring down the assimilation of lipids (fats) by means of the intestinal track. Theanine is an amino corrosive in green tea that can support the arrival of dopamine, the synthetic that makes you "cheerful" and loose. In the event that you have a tendency to eat because of anxiety, this might be helpful. It likewise counters the caffeine so you don't get all jumpy. The ginger added to green tea will enhance processing and include a little flavor-no sugar or drain in this tea!

You will require...

- 1/2 inch of crisp ginger root, peeled and finely hacked OR ½ teaspoon ground ginger

- 1 teaspoon of green tea

- 8 ounces of crisp water

- Raw, natural nectar (discretionary)

Place green tea and ginger in a strainer or sifter and spread with 8 ounces of bubbling water. Soaking green tea for a really long time can abandon it with a severe taste, so don't surpass 3-4 minutes. You can mix in somewhat crude nectar on the off chance that you truly need to sweeten it, however keep away from milk or sugar no matter what. Drink 1-2 glasses every day on a void stomach.

Green Tea for Weight Loss

3. Flower Petal Water

The advantages of flower petal water are sponsored more by narrative proof than anything, yet that is no motivation to disregard this mellow yet reviving beverage. Flower petals go about as an exceptionally delicate diuretic. Diuretics urge your kidneys to put more sodium (salt) into your pee. This abundance salt thus draws water from your blood, diminishing the measure of water in your circulatory framework. This is not "changeless" weight reduction simply water weight-but rather the activity urges you to drink increasingly and keep your framework flushed perfect and hydrated. Staying hydrated, trust it or not, can be tremendously useful to getting thinner.

You will require...

- Handful of new or dried flower petals

- Distilled water (about 1-2 containers)

- A pot with a firmly fitting cover

Note: Be certain, particularly if utilizing new flower petals, that they have not been treated with any kind of concoction (bug sprays, pesticides, herbicides, manures, and so forth.)

Place the pot on the stove, put in the flower petals, and add simply enough refined water to totally cover them. On the off chance that some buoy to the top it's not a major ordeal. Spread the pot with a firmly fitting cover and stew until the petals lose the majority of their shading, around 15-20 minutes.

Strain the fluid into a glass bump and keep in the fridge for up to 6 days. Drink about ½-1 glass each morning on a void stomach.

Rose Water

4. Ginseng

Ginseng is any of 11 perpetual plants with beefy roots fitting in with the type Panax. While there are various types of ginseng, the two that you ought to utilize –also the ones that have had the most controlled twofold visually impaired studies done on them-are American ginseng (Panax quinquefolius) and Asian or Korean ginseng (Panax ginseng.) While generally known as a stimulant to accelerate a drowsy digestion system, that portrayal doesn't do it equity. Ginseng's most noteworthy quality is that it can battle fatigue and help vitality and also mental readiness (in a randomized twofold visually impaired study in 2010 290 disease patients at the Mayo Clinic were given ginseng day by day and it was found to battle even the disabling fatigue brought about by chemotherapy.) This is immense with regards to weight reduction without vitality, it's difficult to exercise. Without exercise, it's close difficult to get thinner in any event healthily. Notwithstanding boosting vitality, there is speculative proof that it can oversee glucose, which influences vitality levels and in addition craving.

You will require...

- 1 teaspoon of hacked American or Korean ginseng

- 8 ounces of new water

- crude nectar/lemon to taste (discretionary)

Generally hack the root and allot 1 teaspoon for some water. Heat water to the point of boiling and after that pour over the ginseng, permitting it to soak for 5-9 minutes. Strain, include nectar or lemon on the off chance that you like, and drink 1-2 times every day.

5. Dandelion and Peppermint

Dandelion and peppermint tea is an awesome beverage that will keep your liver sound. The liver is a mind blowing organ. Not just is it the best way to really detoxify your body, it is additionally assumes a focal part in numerous metabolic procedures a great deal of which influence weight. As far as fat digestion system, the liver is loaded with cells that separate fats and transform them into usable vitality. These cells are likewise in charge of the stream of bile, which helps breakdown and ingest fats. In the digestion system of starches, the liver keeps your glucose relentless, subsequently keeping vitality step up and directing voracity. The rundown goes on, however the fact of the matter is offering your liver offers your weight, as it some assistance with playing a significant part in dealing with some assistance with fatting and their ingestion. Dandelion and peppermint both help your liver. Dandelion has hepatoprotection constituents, with hepatoprotection meaning a capacity to avert harm to the liver. Peppermint and dandelion both naturally empower the creation of bile in the liver, assisting with assimilation and the ingestion of supplements. Combine these two, and you have an effective liver securing tea!

You will require...

- 1 teaspoon of dried dandelion clears out

- 1 teaspoon dried peppermint clears out

- 8 ounces of bubbling water

- Lemon to taste (discretionary)

Pour some bubbling water over the dandelion and peppermint and steep, secured, for 5-10 minutes. Strain, add lemon to taste in the event that you like, and drink a container twice day by day. You can likewise make this with crisp dandelion leaves/roots and new peppermint, simply utilize an unpleasant modest bunch of the new leaves for the sum. In the event that you do use crisp, be totally sure that there have been no chemicals connected to them-this is particularly critical for dandelion. In the event that you utilize dandelion all the time, I propose developing your own.

6. Taste on Sage

We live in a wild world, and the majority of us are pushed around some thing once a day. The thing is, our bodies weren't made to handle consistent anxiety, and it can effectsly affect a wide astypement of capacities including weight pick up/loss. At the point when under anxiety, the body discharges cortisol, a steroid hormone that is a piece of the battle or-flight reaction. Cortisol can impact glucose level (along these lines voracity), and cause vitality to be put away all the more promptly as fat. Neuropeptide Y is a neurochemical that is additionally identified with anxiety. Whenever discharged, it causes development of fat tissue (vitality is put away effortlessly as fat around the belly) and in addition an expansion in hunger. One approach to battle this hidden anxiety can be to ingest more wise, which has quieting consequences for both the body and mind. Making a quieting sage tea, or even simply including it in dishes you cook, is one approach to battle your anxiety levels.

You will require...

- A modest bunch of new sage OR 2 teaspoons of dried sage

- 8 ounces of bubbling water

- Lemon to taste (discretionary)

Pour bubbling water over savvy and soak for 4-5 minutes. Strain, add lemon to taste on the off chance that you like, and drink 1-2 times day by day.

Sage Tea Remedy

7. Bite Gum

Biting gum is an awesome approach to trap your cerebrum (and your stomach) into supposing it's getting more than it is. The kind of the gum decreases hankering and controls the inclination to nibble on something horrible, furthermore empowers the stream of salivation, whose compounds separate starches and fats.

You will require...

- 1 bit of characteristic sugar free gum

Bearings

When you feel the need to begin crunching, pop in a bit of gum.

8. Have a Routine (and stick to it)

Having a routine is, as I would see it, in the main three most essential things you can do to get more fit, straight up there with exercise and count calories. On the off chance that you don't adhere to a normal, you won't get results, and you'll be disheartened. Quite a long while prior I saw a fitness coach and, in the wake of paying a fair whole of cash, I made sense of that it was the routine of going to see her had the greatest effect. It's presumably the single hardest thing you'll do when you attempt to get thinner, however once those propensities get to be hardwired into your cerebrum, things will just get less demanding.

9. Simply Add Water

Staying hydrated is an imperative part of weight reduction that individuals frequently get over you would prefer not to put on water weight and feel bloated right? Either that or you hear that you ought to drink super cold water to smolder more calories. Not precisely. The thought that super cold water smolders more calories on the grounds that your body tries to "warm it up" first might actually be genuine, yet the impact is miniscule (like 8 calories miniscule.) Rather, you should be hydrated for your body to run easily, and that incorporates blazing fat. It flushes terrible stuff through your framework, furthermore checks hunger. What's more, don't fuss about water weight-in the event that you are staying hydrated, your body is more averse to hold water since it essentially doesn't have the need to-like how eating more can make weight reduction less demanding, inside of reason. I ought to additionally say-DO NOT BUY INTO SPECIALTY WATERS! Get your vitamins through your eating routine or supplements. Those waters are worse for you truth be told some are so stacked with seasoning and what not they match pop.

You will require...

- 8 ounces of new water

Drink no less than some new water each day.

10. Coconut Oil (as a substitution fat)

In the 1970's and '80's, soaked fats got pushed into the spotlight as the fundamental driver for obesity. Coconut oil, being an immersed fat, was hurled alongside whatever is left of them. The more advantageous option that we made? Trans-fat. One could say that exploded backward a small piece eh? Coconut oil isn't only any old immersed fat however; it contains remarkable fats called medium chain triglycerides that offer you some assistance with using vitality (otherwise known as calories) all the more effectively. MCT's are in reality an immersed fat, yet they are not the same the same number of the other soaked fats we find out about those fats are long chain triglycerides. Why does the length make a difference? Its compound cosmetics is the thing that decides how our body forms it and separates it. MCT's are not separated in the digestion systems, and along these lines don't escape quickly as fat. Rather, they assimilated in place and sent right to the liver, where they are utilized as vitality. Presently lounging around eating coconut oil isn't going to make you get more fit, however utilizing it as a substitution fat can be a decent decision. Notwithstanding that, out and out coconut oil is an unfathomable craving suppressant (it's verging on alarming, really.) Tack on that it can raise vitality levels and you will probably get out, move around, and exercise.

Similarly as studies on it go, here are some that I said in The Everyday Roots Book. In 2002 the Journal of Nutrition presumed that it can help weight reduction when utilized as a part of spot of long chain triglycerides. It was additionally appeared to firmly check hunger and it seemed to build the smoldering of calories. In 2003 Obesity Research found that it might blaze calories, most likely because of the way that it helped vitality. In 2010 the International Journal of Food Sciences and Nutrition additionally found that it could help digestion system and decrease craving.

You will require...

- 2 tablespoons of good virgin icy squeezed coconut oil

Twice every day, take 1 tablespoon of coconut oil. You can take it some time recently, amid, or after a feast. On the off chance that you tend to battle with extents, I recommend taking it before you eat, or if treat is your evil spirit, take it directly after supper. As far as substitution I've utilized it as a part of spot of olive oil and cherish it.

Coconut Oil Helps You Lose Weight

11. Plain Yogurt and Honey

This is a great breakfast/nibble. It's one of those "I wouldn't figure this is beneficial for me!" write nourishments. The probiotics in yogurt do ponders for the digestive track and keeps up a sound parity of gut greenery that advances absorption and the breakdown of specific substances (such as fat.) When you digestive track is running easily, your body is preparing things better and it's not as prone to pack on the pounds. The nectar is only a little included (sound) sweetness to fulfill any yearnings you may have. The wonderful thing here is that you truly don't feel like you're getting shorted any flavor or totality when you eat it. For ideal weight reduction amazingness, attempt low fat yogurt.

Note: There was at one time a period when certain substantial organizations started to add such a great amount of sugar to their yogurt the sums surpassed those found in sugary breakfast grain, as Lucky Charms. Individuals were eating it up and thinking about how it could be so divine and bravo, when truly the picture and wholesomeness of yogurt was essentially being mishandled. Perused the nourishment mark first.

You will require...

- 1/2-1 measure of plain (not vanilla) yogurt

- 1 tablespoon of natural crude nectar, or to taste

Eat this for a nibble or breakfast, including the nectar for flavor. Don't hesitate to have a go at including new organic product or even oats for a little astypement.

Yogurt and Honey

12. Get Enough Sleep

Our body is a strong unit, a mind boggling framework, not simply singular parts. Everything must be working congruously for things to be adjusted and revise like your weight. Thinks about have demonstrated that even only a smidgen of lack of sleep over the brief span edge of 4 evenings results in expanded insulin resistance, and basically ages the digestion system 10-20 years in that time period. The fat cells affectability to insulin dropped by 30% to levels normally found in individuals who were fat or diabetic. By getting the perfect measure of rest, you're accomplishing more than simply resting your body-you're guaranteeing that all frameworks are go, and that you have the most obvious opportunity conceivable to succeed at shedding pounds.

13. Dark Pepper and Lemon Juice

This fiery little invention contains dark pepper and lemon juice to make a beverage that can offer you some assistance with keeping ahead on your weight reduction fight. Dark pepper contains an actually happening concoction compound called piperine, which is in charge of giving it its impactful flavor. A few new studies have demonstrated that piperine can meddle with the qualities that control the era of fat cells, and also diminishing fat levels in the circulation system and improving the retention of supplements from our nutritions. Lemon juice can help in absorption and give your G.I. track some assistance with regards to separating nourishments.

You will require...

- Several sprinkles of newly ground dark pepper

- Juice of a large portion of a lemon

- Fresh water

Blend lemon juice with water and sprinkle in dark pepper (around 3-4 turns of the pepper processor.) Drink once every day after a dinner.

Lemon and Black Pepper Drink

14. Bottle Gourd Juice

Bottle gourds are old-world hard-shelled natural products that recounted proof proposes can offer you some assistance with losing weight. Individuals who swear by it find that, because of its high fiber content, it causes a buzz of totality and checks hankering. It likewise has high water content (dependably something to be thankful for) and has various extraordinary supplements. On the off chance that you do choose to drink bottle gourd juice, don't do as such in a manner that you utilize it to "starve" yourself (see underneath.) Your body needs all the (great) nourishment and supplements it needs to keep up an adjusted eating routine, in any case, it's an incredible approach to oppose longings and potential nibbling sprees!

You will require...

- some jug gourd juice, chilled

- A little lime juice

Headings

When you feel the inclination to nibble, drink a glass of icy jug gourd juice with a dash of lime juice included.

15. Eat More (and make sense of why you're eating in any case)

Hardship never works. It is an excruciating battle that will quite often bring about disappointment. Rather than keeping your body from the supplements it needs to stay solid, eat "all the more" well done. Separate your suppers to 5 or 6 little ones a day to lessen eating (which is the point at which a decent lump of weight addition happens for many people) and to keep your body from putting away more fat-which is does when it feels "starved." Also ask yourself for what reason you're eating in any case we so frequently eat out of fatigue or nerves or stretch. Hold up until you feel a thunder and let your stomach let you know when it needs to eat.

16. Apple Snacks

An apple a day keeps the weight under control! While not flooding with supplements such as different natural products or vegetables, apples still have various advantages that can add to weight reduction. In the first place, they are stuffed with fiber, which checks voracity, so eat one when you feel the inclination to nibble on some less-attractive nourishments. Second, they can control glucose levels, and thusly manage your hunger and vitality levels. Third, the pectin in apples can bring down cholesterol, and serve as another approach to direct glucose, by abating the retention of sugars. At last, apples are a normally low-sodium nourishment, which can forestall abundance water maintenance and water weight.

You will require...

- 1-2 crisp apples

Flush and cut an apple, and eat one to two day by day. Leave the skin on, as that contains a decent measure of fiber.

Apples

17. Include More Asparagus

Pay consideration on regular foods grown from the ground, and jump on the asparagus when it tags along. Asparagus is supplement thick and, similar to apples, contains a great deal of fiber to control craving. It additionally contains a large group of vitamins that cooperate to metabolize blood glucose, in this manner manage glucose. On the off chance that you wind up feeling puffy or bloated, asparagus is a mellow diuretic that can lessen bloating and abandon you feeling your best. Have a go at eating asparagus steamed in favor of your most loved dishes-this vegetable needn't bother with much to make it taste great

You will require...

- 1 bundle of asparagus

- some water

Headings

Wash the asparagus and softly peel the stems in the event that they are thick. Place in a container with ½-1 inch of water, and cover with a firmly fitting top. Turn the warmth to medium high and steam for 3 minutes, or until the asparagus is delicate and can be punctured effortlessly with a fork.

Asparagus

18. Put Your Fork or Spoon Down Between Bites

Your mind lingers behind your stomach by around 20 minutes, which ,implies that it isn't the best thing to depend on with regards to telling your when you're full. To stay away from over-eating, and in this manner devouring additional un-required calories, moderate down your eating by putting your fork or spoon down between chomps. You may feel somewhat senseless at in the first place, yet it can truly cause with regards to dealing with your weight.

19. Nibble on Flax

Flax seed has been known not with digestive illnesses for a considerable length of time, and this runs as one with weight reduction. Flax seeds are high in fiber, and in addition adhesive, which brings down cholesterol. It has likewise been demonstrated to lower glucose levels. With such a high measure of fiber, flax seeds additionally go about as a characteristic tender approach to control solid discharges and advance sound gut microorganisms, both which function admirably to offer you some assistance with managing weight. It is imperative to eat flaxseed ground, as it tends to go through the digestive track undigested if eaten entire, in this manner denying you of its healthful advantages.

You will require...

- 1 tablespoon of ground flaxseed

Once every day eat a tablespoon of ground flaxseed-sprinkling it over grain or oats if my own inclination.

20. Milk Thistle

Milk thorn contains dynamic flavonoid mixes all things considered known as simirilyn. Simalrilyn secures the liver which is an imperative organ with regards to overseeing weight and empowering weight reduction. At the point when your liver is impeded and lazy, weight reduction can be eased back by up to 30%*. The simarilyn in milk thorn can switch this. There are a few approaches to take milk thorn, be that as it may I suggest a case structure (ensure the source is solid) or as a tincture, since milk thorn does not give its advantages when saturated with water, (for example, when made into a tea.)

You will require...

- Milk thorn cases or tincture

Take after

on the bundling for measurement.

21. Proceed, Eat That Chocolate

Keep in mind hardship barely works? When you get the inclination for a sweet treat, swing to dim chocolate. It will check your longing on account of its insulin-resistance bringing down flavonoids. The solid fats in dim chocolate can likewise moderate the assimilation of sugar into your circulation system, counteracting "insulin spikes." Studies have demonstrated that eating some can put a stop to desires for sugar, salt, and fat. Be that as it may, the chocolate must be 70% cocoa, else it has an excessive amount of milk or sugar added to be valuable.

You will require...

- 70% dull chocolate

Specifically after a feast, eat a bit of dim chocolate generally the measure of your thumb to gather its advantages.

Dim Chcolate

22. Join the Navy... Beans

Beans, beans, the otherworldly organic product, the more you eat the more you... get in shape? Obviously, since the protein in naval force beans can take a while to process, thusly diminishing hankering and helping in weight reduction administration. The fiber in naval force beans can likewise bring down cholesterol.

You will require...

- 1 measure of dried naval force beans

- some water

Set up the naval force beans by including some new water to a pot for some dried beans, so that the fluid level is around 1-2 inches about the beans. Heat the water to the point of boiling and after that decrease to a stew, halfway covering the pot. Skim off any froth that creates, and stew for 1 to 1 ½ hours until delicate. Add to a plate of mixed greens or appreciate as a dish all alone.

When you're attempting to make sense of how to get in shape, realize that there truly is no enchantment thing that works for everybody. Yes, eating routine and exercise are essential, however individuals are distinctive, bodies are distinctive, and you need to consider things, for example, hereditary qualities, wellbeing conditions, sexual orientation, and age. You may be scowling at your collaborator chowing down on doughnuts at the workplace while you pick at a plate of mixed greens and think about how they figure out how to stay so fit when they eat whatever they need however don't let this drag you down. The trip is distinctive for everybody, except there is dependably an approach to finish it. Also, if all else fails, disentangle the circumstance eat great nourishment, get appropriate exercise. We've transformed eating and weight reduction into a science that dives into such infinitesimal things we have a feeling that we aren't equipped for eating right or getting in shape without expert help. Expecting you have no remarkable condition that convolutes the circumstance, you can achieve your objectives all alone! It might be troublesome, however hey, that is the place things like these cures can loan some assistance.

Tips

- Weight isn't all that matters. Muscle weighs more than fat, and being fit and sound is more essential than being unfathomably "thin." Healthy looks great on you, and keep in mind it!

- Never disparage stress as a reason for weight pick up. The body can't perform any capacity, including blazing fat for vitality, ideally when under anxiety.

- There are no super-nourishments. Try not to depend on one thing to offer you some assistance with losing weight-dependably keep up an adjusted eating routine.

- Don't eat before bed. Your digestion system hammers on the brakes when you go to rest, so eating around evening time makes weight increase intense to maintain a strategic distance from.

- Get a pal to make objectives that you two endeavor towards. When you lose determination or inspiration, a companion can be every one of that stands in the middle of progress and difficulty.

- Read a book called Salt, Sugar, Fat: How the Food Giants Hooked Us In by New York Times investigative journalist Michael Moss. Take care of business. It will give you something new and unmistakable to clutch when you are attempting to dodge garbage nourishment. At the danger of sounding cheesy, it really changed my life.

cheerful, you really shine from inside out.

Herbs for Obesity

- Along the lines of the first tip-deal with your weight to be solid, and at last, cheerful. Disregard pictures of impeccable figures. Disregard the senseless things society shells you with, letting you know what you ought to resemble. To say that is simpler said than done is the modest representation of the truth of the century, yet do attempt to remember it. When you are sound, and

Aloe Vera (Aloe barbadensis)

Aloe vera juice enhances processing and washes down the digestive tract.

(Astragalus gummifer)

Astragalus expands vitality and enhances supplement ingestion.

Honey bee dust

Honey bee dust empowers the digestion system and checks longing. Take up to 1 teaspoon day by day.

Bladderwrack (Fucus vesiculosus)

Bladderwrack contain iodine, which upgrades thyroid capacity. Dose: Take 150 milligrams at breakfast and another 150 milligrams lunch for two months.

Alert: Check with your specialist before taking this herb in the event that you have a thyroid issue, hypertension, or heart issues. On the off chance that you are adversely affected by shellfish and/or touchy to iodine, don't take this herb. Likewise don't take kelp and bladderwrack in the meantime.

Brewer's yeast

Brewer's yeast will decrease different desires for nourishment and drink.

Chickweed (Stellaria media)

This herb an incredible people notoriety for shedding weight.

You can eat it crude in plates of mixed greens. Then again, you can steam it and eat it like a vegetable. For an incredible weight reduction plate of mixed greens, blend chickweed, dandelion, evening primrose, stinging bramble (cooked and cooled), plantain and purslane. Add this to your standard plate of mixed greens.

Coconut oil

Coconut oil, separated from coconuts, is a rich hotspot for medium chain triglycerides. Medium chain triglycerides (MCTS) are extraordinary types of soaked fats isolated out from coconut oil that range long from six to twelve carbon chains. Dissimilar to general fats, MCTs don't seem to bring about weight pick up; they really advance weight reduction.

Medium Chain Triglycerides and Long Chain Triglycerides

Medium chain triglycerides (MCTS) are unique types of immersed fats isolated out from coconut oil. It range long from six to twelve carbon chains.

The long-chain triglycerides (LCTS) are the most plentiful fats found in nature. LCTs are the capacity fat for both people and plants. They run long from eighteen to twenty-four carbons.

MCTs are utilized by the body uniquely in contrast to LCTs. This is a direct result of the distinction long of carbon chains. The bigger LCTs are troublesome for the body to metabolize. So the body tends to store these fats. MCTS, then again, are anything but difficult to metabolize. Along these lines, they are quickly smoldered as vitality. They likewise advance the blazing of LCTs.

As a result of the way body handles MCTs, MCTs don't seem to bring about weight increase like the traditional fats do. They, truth be told, really advance weight reduction. LCTs are normally put away in the fat stores. Following their vitality is preserved, a high fat eating regimen diminishes the metabolic rate. Bring down the digestion system, higher the weight pick up.

Researchers propose that medium-Chain Triglycerides advance weight reduction by expanding thermogenesis (heat creation). Thermogenesis is the system by which the body "squanders" calories. There is confirmation that the level of eating routine affected thermogenesis is the thing that figures out if an individual is prone to be overweight. In incline people, a feast might animate up to a forty-percent expansion in warmth creation. Conversely, overweight people regularly encounter just a ten-percent or less increment in warmth generation. The nutrition vitality is put away as opposed to being changed over to warm. In reality, the nutrition is all the more effectively changed over if there should arise an occurrence of LCTs. In this way, ther eis less requirement for them to acquire the same vitality. (LCTs is similar to a fuel effective auto. It needs less fuel to go to the same separation when contrasted with a fuel swallowing auto (like MCTs). Along these lines, for the same nutrition utilization, LCTs will have more fat put away int he body advancing weight pick up.

This has been exhibited in clinical trials.

In one study, researchers looked at the thermogenic impact of a fatty eating routine containing forty-percent fat as MCTs to that of one containing forty-percent fat as LCTs.

The thermogenic impact (calories squandered six hours after a feast) of the MCTs was twice as extraordinary as that of the LCTs. (120 calories versus 66 calories.) It gives the idea that the abundance vitality gave by fats as MCTs would not be effectively put away as fat. Rather, they would be blazed and create heat.

A subsequent study exhibited that MCT oil given over a six-day period can increment diet-actuated thermogenesis by fifty percent.

In another study, scientists gave single suppers of 400 calories made altogether out of either MCTs or LTCs. Six hours in the wake of eating, researchers found that the thermogeneic impact of MCTs was three times more noteworthy than that of LCTs. Interestingly, MCTs had no impact on the blood fat level. The LCTs, then again, raised blood fat levels by sixty eight percent. Blood fat level is a noteworthy danger element for contracting CHDs.

Scientists inferred that substituting MCTs for LCTs in your eating regimen would deliver weight reduction the length of the calorie level continued as before.

Keeping in mind the end goal to pick up the advantage from MCTs, an eating routine must stay low in LCTs. Use MCTs (coconut oil or different items containing MCTs) as an oil for plate of mixed greens dressing, as a bread spread, or basically taken as a supplement. Coconut oil is a critical herb utilized as a part of Ayurvedic Medicine. Ayurvedic doctors regularly recommend that coconut oil be rubbed on the body.

Prescribed Dosage: 1 to 2 tablespoons for each day.

Dandelion (Taraxacum officinale)

Dandelion might flush out the kidneys, support digestion system, and off-set a longing for desserts. Eat the leaves crude in a plate of mixed greens or make a tea by bubbling 2 to 3 tsp of the root in some water for I 0 to 15 minutes. Drink three times each day.

Evening primrose (Oenothera biennis).

This herb is a decent hotspot for tryptophan which is accepted to help in weight reduction. Take a half-teaspoon of night primrose oil three times each day.

Fennel (Foeniculum vulgare)

Fennel expels bodily fluid and fat from the intestinal tract, and is a characteristic longing suppressant.

Fenugreek (Trigonella foenum-graecum)

Fenugreek is helpful for dissolving fat inside of the liver.

Green Tea (Camellia sinensis)

Green tea improves the capacity of the body to smolder fat. Pick an institutionalized concentrate containing 50 percent catechin and 90 percent downright polyphenols and take 300 milligrams thirty minutes before breakfast and an additional thirty minutes before lunch. Try not to take more.

Guggul (Commiphora mukul)

This is a prominent herb utilized as a part of Ayurveda. Guggul is as often as possible prescribed by Ayurveda experts for weight control notwithstanding use in bringing down cholesterol. In clinical trials, admission of guggul subsidiaries consistently for three months results in four times the weight reduction contrasted with fake treatment.

Measurements: 2.25 grams twice every day

Kelp (Fucus spp.)

Kelp is a kind of ocean growth that is rich in cell reinforcement vitamins and iodine. It is accepted to animate a hormone created by the thyroid organ that is in charge of boosting digestion system, so you'll blaze more calories by the hour. You can likewise get different types of kelp in your adding so as to eat routine them to soups and servings of mixed greens. Kelp is extremely helpful for thyroid-related obesity.

Measurement: Take 300-1,500 mg every day as coordinated on the mark.

Alert: Check with your specialist before taking kelp in the event that you have a thyroid issue, hypertension, or heart issues.

Licorice (Glycyrrhiza glabra)

Licorice root reinforces the adrenal organs, in this manner maintaining a controlled glucose level and diminish desires for desserts. Licorice tastes sweet.

Measurement: Take a measure of licorice day by day, one week out of consistently for up to three months. Licorice can likewise be added to different teas to sweeten them.

Alert: Do not take licorice independent from anyone else every day for over five days on end, as it can hoist circulatory strain. Try not to take it at all on the off chance that you have hypertension. This herb ought to be utilized with alert. Check the home grown database for other critical wellbeing data.

Malabar tamarind (Gareinia cantbogia)

The Malabar tamarind is a yellowish organic product that is about the extent of an orange, with a meager skin and profound wrinkles like an oak seed squash. It is local to southern India, where it is dried and utilized widely as a part of curries (particularly angle). It looks dark when dried.

The dried product of Malabar Tamarind contains around thirty percent hydroxycitric corrosive. It is an intense lipogenic inhibitor. (Lipogenic inhibitor is a substance which keeps the creation of fat.)

In creature ponders, hydroxycitrate has been appeared to be an effective inhibitor of fat development. One study demonstrated that hydroxycitrate delivered a "critical lessening in nourishment allow, and body weight pick up" in rats. The outcomes in people are not yet demonstrated.

Notwithstanding hindering the generation of fat, hydroxycitrate might likewise smother ravenousness.

Note that hydroxycitrate just restrains the change of starches into fat. It will have no impact if a high-fat eating regimen is expended.

Prescribed Dosage: 500 mg three times each day. Bring it alongside a supplement of Chromium for best results.

Pineapple (Ananas comosus)

Pineapple contains a compound called bromelain, which processes both proteins and fats.

Cultivator Dr. Duke reported that one individual in Costa Rica lost 100 pounds by eating one entire new pineapple for each day. Pineapple is stacked with nutrition, and is likewise awesome for your processing.

Plantain or psyllium (Plantago)

Psyllium is the seed of Plantain. Metamucil is a business item that contain psyllium.

Cultivators say that the weight reduction impact of plantain and psyllium is identified with the springy fiber (adhesive) in the seeds and to particular chemicals (polyphenols) in the takes off.

In one Italian study, researchers gave ladies who were truly fat (more than 60 percent over their prescribed weight) three grams of plantain in water 30 minutes before dinners. The plantain bunch lost more weight than a comparable gathering of ladies who just cut back on their eating routine.

Dosage: Take a teaspoonful of psyllium blended well with milk.

Some other important herbs

#1 Turmeric

Most normally connected with Indian nutrition, turmeric has been appeared to decrease aggravation, elevated amounts of which might be a noteworthy reason for obesity and trouble getting more fit.

#2 Cinnamon

Generously sprinkling cinnamon on your oats can control your glucose and insulin levels, shielding you from diabetes while at the same time dealing with your craving.

#3 Cayenne pepper

A compound in hot peppers called dihydrocapsiate has been appeared to expand the body's capacity to smolder fat when eaten three times each day.

#4 Ginger

New or powdered ginger might have the capacity to decrease your ravenousness and cut yearnings.

#5 Black Pepper

The substance in dark pepper that gives it that peppery flavor, called piperine, has been appeared to offer the body some assistance with burning more calories through the procedure of thermogenesis. Piperine can likewise offer your body some assistance with using supplements all the more productively.

#6 Coriander

Coriander is a typical fixing in the Indian zest blends that have been appeared to increment metabolic capacity and uplift weight reduction in creature contemplates.

#7 Cumin

Correspondingly, in spite of the fact that it hasn't been concentrated on independent from anyone else, cumin has been appeared to enhance weight reduction when blended with different herbs and flavors.

#8 Parsley

A few studies that took a gander at rats have demonstrated that parsley can lessen the measure of glucose present in the blood. On the off chance that this is valid in people, parsley would likely control voracity and advance solid preparing of nourishment into vitality.

#9 Ginseng

Different creature ponders have demonstrated that the herb panax ginseng can help in weight diminishment, and even moderate weight pick up coming about because of eating regimens high in fat.

#10 Cardamom

Concentrates on in rats have demonstrated that cardamom can help in bringing down blood glucose and directing insulin, and additionally bringing down levels of LDL (terrible) cholesterol.

#11 Cloves

In the same way as other of alternate flavors on this rundown, cloves can offer you some assistance with speeding so as to lose weight up your digestion system and helping your body to smolder more calories.

#12 Mustard

Mustard seed appears to have a thermogenic impact on the body, making it smolder more calories as it summaries nutrition. Past the mustard you may connect with franks, take a stab at flavoring your nourishment with powdered dry mustard seed for an additional kick!

#13 Garlic

Adding garlic to your nutrition in crisp or powdered structure may have the capacity to offer you some assistance with metabolizing starches and fats all the more proficiently. Creature ponders have appeared that garlic might keep the body from making more fat.

#14 Green Tea

Green tea is well-demonstrated to have various medical advantages. Notwithstanding anticipating disease and diabetes, green tea can likewise accelerate your digestion system and offer you some assistance with losing weight.

#15 Peppermint

A study distributed in 2009 found that the odor of peppermint can diminish craving. In the study, members who spent a week noticing peppermint before they ate by and large expended 1,800 less calories during the time than the control bunch.

On the off chance that you need to get more fit, you know the best way to guarantee sound advance and changing so as to endure achievement is the means by which you eat and expanding your movement level. In any case, there are various herbs that can help this excursion along, whether by helping so as to accelerate your fat-blazing digestion system or you smother desires.

These main 5 herbs can quicken your body's common capacity to dispose of muscle to fat ratio ratios both securely and successfully:

Some special herbs for weight loss

1. Hoodia Gordonii

Hoodia made genuine additions in ubiquity a couple of years prior amid which time its advantageous properties turned out to be all the more surely understood by the overall population. Presently, the dust has settled a bit, however unadulterated Hoodia is still a viable weight reduction help with genuine support. Utilized by seekers as a part of desert locales of Africa, the herb lessens longings and permits you to cut calories without sentiments of hardship. Since there are numerous weight reduction helps conveying the Hoodia name, be careful that what you are getting is the genuine article.

2. Damiana

This is a wild bush local toward the West Indies, Mexico, and Central America. It has an astypement of employments, however most as of late has been promoted as a weight reduction help. This could be a direct result of its consequences for the digestive framework, once in a while empowering free stools and the ensuing loss of water weight. Then again, a promising study demonstrated that when matched with different herbs, Damiana deferred gastric exhausting, giving a feeling of completion to a more drawn out period subsequent to eating [1].

3. Gymnema

This herb is local to Africa and has been utilized for quite a long time as a part of Ayurvedic medication. It is said to adjust glucose levels and is regularly suggested for individuals experiencing diabetes. It is said to square sugar assimilation and stop sugar longings, a noteworthy benefactor to a few individuals' weight issues.

4. Kelp

Kelp is rich in iodine, a substance that can help in weight reduction. A critical iodine lack can really prompt hypothyroidism – a condition that has been connected to weight pick up. Notwithstanding assisting with weight reduction, kelp controls thyroid capacity.

5. Green Coffee Bean

In opposition to what you might at first think, the weight reduction advantages of green espresso bean don't originate from caffeine, and it is not a stimulant. A characteristic compound in green espresso bean called chlorogenic, in any case, has been appeared to increment fat assimilation and stop weight pick up. An investigation of green espresso bean separate distributed in the Diabetes, Metabolic Syndrome and Obesity Journal demonstrated those supplementing with green espresso bean lost a normal of 17 pounds over a 12 week period [2].

The way to weight reduction is appropriate eating routine and exercise. Herbs can supplement this solid way of life. A weight reduction solution or over the counter stimulant can contain obscure and conceivably destructive fixings, yet amazing herbals can be very worthwhile when acquired from the right source.

Herbs are what are characteristic and you can extremely well take help of these herbs for weight reduction. Have you ever thought why individuals in the past were not all that worried about getting fat? Why obesity was not an issue as it is today? From the time onwards when individuals began preparing common nourishments and driving life which needs physical developments, they likewise began putting on weight. Indeed, even today on the off chance that you converse with somebody who has shed pounds, you'll be recounted heaps of herbs and characteristic nourishments alongside exercises that had offered them in losing some assistance with weighting. In this way, why not you too think about the top herbs for weight reduction. Just knowing is insufficient. Follow up on this. Receive these home grown solutions for weight reduction and get fit as a fiddle not in a flash but rather with enduring impact!

1. Green Tea for Weight Loss

Green tea is stacked with cancer prevention agents as well as has thermo-genic properties inside of itself. Thermogenesis can be comprehended as the procedure of warmth generation in life forms including people. It builds utilization of vitality and fat oxidation so you smolder your muscle to fat quotients speedier. Green tea likewise feels you full so you don't eat more than you require. Not just this, EGCG in green tea diminishes the measure of fat that your body assimilates when you eat your nourishment. This is useful in your weight reduction endeavors as well as in decreasing your cholesterol level.

How to have green tea for weight reduction?

Make your green tea by setting 1-2 tsp of good quality green tea in a container or dish. Pour boiling point water over it and let it mix for a moment. Taste it. In the event that it is not sufficiently solid for your taste buds, let it blend for one more moment and afterward taste once more. Continue tasting each moment to comprehend what quality of green tea would you incline toward. At that point onwards, you might mix your tea for that numerous minutes. Typically individuals blend green tea for 2-

5 minutes. Strain and drink some green tea. As this is for weight reduction, its attractive not to add any sweetener to the tea.

Have green tea rather than general tea or espresso in the morning. It has enough caffeine to begin off your day. Likewise, this will accelerate your digestion system right in the morning so you might smolder more calories for the duration of the day.

Drink no less than 4 some green tea for the duration of the day. This will offer you some assistance with feeling full and you'll focus lesser on gorging. Having some green tea before or after dinners is a smart thought.

2. Ginseng for Weight Loss

Ginseng has long been utilized by Chinese medication as a conventional prescription for vitality, stamina, and general prosperity. Current specialists have additionally observed ginseng to be powerful for weight reduction and in addition diabetes control. One of the looks into discusses ginseng's capacity to make body cells lesser fit for putting away fat. Ginseng is an adaptogen, a substance which enhances the body's ability to adapt to physical, passionate and natural anxiety. You can discover ginseng in new and also dried structure. While now and then leaves of ginseng plant are additionally included with its root yet the root is the most advantageous part of this plant. Ginseng can offer you in two approaches to lose some assistance with weighting. To begin with, it will help your digestion system wherein when you eat, you will store less fat when contrasted with when you don't take ginseng. Also, ginseng will fill you with vitality so you stay more dynamic and in this manner spend more calories.

Make ginseng tea for weight reduction

Dried ginseng root-4 tbsp

Water-4 mugs

Nectar (discretionary)- 1-2 tsp

Cinnamon (discretionary)- ¼ – ½ tsp

Do this:

Heat up the water in a container.

Add ginseng root to the bubbling water.

Stew for 60 minutes.

Expel from the warmth and strain.

Include nectar and/or cinnamon. Nectar diminishes the astringent persistent flavor f ginseng herb and cinnamon powder can make it somewhat sweet-smelling.

Drink one glass each in the morning and after lunch.

3. Guggul Herb Extract for Weight Loss

Guggul is an age old home grown prescription suggested by Ayurveda for different wellbeing conditions including weight reduction. Furthermore, additionally essential is that advanced studies have likewise upheld the impact of guggul herb in weight reduction. Guggul gum sap is separated from the Commiphora mukul tree or the mukul myrrh tree. Gum guggul separate contains guggulsterone, a plant steroid which is thought to be hostile to tumor, against angiogenic and cholesterol-bringing down segment. On the other hand, the weight reduction impact of guggul originates from its movement on thyroid organ. Thyroid hormones are key for accurate metabolic rate which chooses the amount of calories would you smolder in a day. As guggul animates thyroid capacity, your metabolic rate goes to the ideal level and weight reduction gets to be less demanding and speedier. The included preferences of guggul are brought down cholesterol levels and a decent state of mind as well. Furthermore, in light of the fact that, it doesn't fortify your focal sensory system, it is a protected herb for weight reduction.

Approaches to assume guggul for weight reduction

Guggul concentrate is effortlessly accessible in type of tablets in wellbeing stores, particularly Ayurveda natural medications stores. By and large, you ought to take 75 milligrams of guggul concentrate isolated in 3 measurements. This implies 25 milligrams as one measurement. Now and then 100 milligrams can likewise be taken however it's ideal to counsel an Ayurvedic specialist or a cultivator before you take guggul supplement.

In the event that you choose to take guggul gum, you might keep 1 gram (about ¼ tsp) of this sap under your tongue or inside your mouth with the goal that it breaks down there. Do it 4 times each day.

4. Hibiscus Tea for Weight Loss

The delightful blossoms of Hibiscus are stacked with supplements, flavonoids and different minerals. The amylase inhibitors in this herb help in bringing down retention of fats and sugars. The fats and sugars in your body are separated by hibiscus with the goal that they can be flushed out of body. Hibiscus blossoms additionally have gentle diuretic property s, which o that you shed water weight as well and decrease your bloating. Your body gets included favorable position of fortified insusceptibility because of the cancer prevention agents present hibiscus.

How to make hibiscus tea for weight reduction?

Hibiscus tea can be served icy and additionally hot. Frosty hibiscus tea takes more opportunity to be made than the more sweltering one.

Make chilly hibiscus tea

Get this:

Dry hibiscus blossoms 1 glass

Water-8 containers

Nectar (discretionary)- according to taste

Do this:

Get new hibiscus blossoms, the ones that are going to sprout.

Separate the petals and place them on a paper. Abandon them for couple of days to get dry.

Once dried, take one measure of dried hibiscus bloom petals.

Absorb them the water for around 1-2 days or till the time they blur away.

Strain and store in fridge. They can be put away in ice chest for around 5 days.

When you need to drink this hibiscus tea, take a glass from the entire part and add nectar to this. You might likewise include different fixings like cinnamon or lemon juice to give it some more taste.

In the event that you need to have hot tea, warm this icy hibiscus tea on stove top or in a microwave broiler. You might likewise make hot hibiscus tea through other system portrayed underneath.

Make hot hibiscus tea

Get this:

Dried hibiscus petals-2 tbsp

Water-2 mugs

Nectar (discretionary)- according to taste

Do this:

Place water in a pot and add the hibiscus petals to it.

Heat to the point of boiling and after that stew for 5-10 minutes.

Strain and include nectar if necessary. You might likewise include lemon, cinnamon and so on.

Make the most of your hot hibiscus tea a get in shape!

Precautionary measure: If you are a pregnant or nursing lady or taking some pharmaceutical, counsel your specialist before taking any home grown tea including hibiscus tea.

5. Yerba Mate for Weight Loss

Yerba Mate is a conventional South American drink. It is indeed an implantation made with dried and matured yerba mate plant and which is inebriated in parties from a solitary gourd and bombilla. Because of its medical advantages, this beverage has come to be known as tea notwithstanding when it has more likenesses to espresso. Generally as espresso can stimulate you because of its caffeine content, yerba mate can likewise top you off with stamina again because of its caffeine. The distinction is that yerba mate will likewise build the rate at which your body smolders calories. Aside from expanding your metabolic rate, yerba mate additionally gives you the advantages of diverse vitamins, minerals, amino acids and cell reinforcements. It additionally helps in backing off your assimilation with the goal that you feel more full for more and expend less calories amid the day. In this way, it bodes well to supplant your morning espresso with yerba mate tea for weight reduction!

How to make yerba mate tea for weight reduction?

While socially an exceptional gourd (likewise called a mate) and a bombilla (metal straw with an empty sifted base) is utilized to imbue yerba mate and to drink it, you might utilize a French press (espresso press) to make your yerba mate tea. All things considered, you are not drinking yerba mate for social reason but rather for extremely individual reason, for your weight reduction!

Get this:

Dried yerba mate herb – 1 tbsp

Hot (not bubbling) water-1-2 containers

Do this:

Place dried yerba mate herb (around 1 tbsp) at the base of your espresso press.

Include 1 some high temp water (not bubbling water) to this.

Mix a little and spread. Leave the plunger up on to your French press. The espresso press permits space for leaves to imbue and grow completely. The powdered little particles additionally get sifted through its fine strainer.

Let steep for 3-5 minutes.

Pour in your container and appreciate.

In the event that this appears a great deal to do, implant your yerba mate in fillable teabags.

6. Pu-erh Tea for Weight Loss

Getting its name from the town of Pu-erh in China where it was initially developed 2000 years back, this is yet another inexplicable herb for weight reduction. This Chinese tea invigorates your spleen and makes it sound which can then process and ingest nourishment supplements well alongside flushing out unreasonable body liquid. It supports your digestion system with the goal that you can blaze more fat and that too at speedier rate.

Tips to drink Pu-erh tea for weight reduction

There is set time to drink this natural tea for weight reduction. On the off chance that you drink it at different times, it might bring about weight pick up. You might drink this tea following 1 hour of your dinners. This bodies to take out all the fat that has not yet been assimilated.

There are two types of pu-erh-crude and ready. Both are useful for weight reduction. In any case, crude pu-erh works speedier yet might invigorate your stomach more than required. To secure your stomach, aged pu-erh is great. What you can do is to have both the teas to accomplish a sound weight reduction. Drink matured pu-erh tea in the morning; crude pu-erh tea after early afternoon feast; and aged pu-erh after dinner.

In the event that it is totally for weight reduction reason, attempt to supplant every one of your beverages with Pu-erh tea. Savor it spot of your teas, espressos even soups!

How to make pu-erh tea?

Get this:

Pu-erh tea leaves-½ – 1 tsp

Heated water-1-2 glasses

Do this:

Place pu-erh tea it in a teapot.

Pour somewhat boiling hot water over it to wash off with the goal that you might uproot any polluting influences. Dispose of the water.

Pour boiling point water over the flushed tea.

Let steep for 2 minutes.

Strain and drink.

7. Grapefruit for Weight Loss

An examination directed in Canada has found a fat smoldering atom in the exceptionally solid grapefruit. A flavonoid is available in grapefruit which is called Naringenin. This part adjusts the glucose levels in your body and avoids metabolic disorder which can make you fat. This can likewise give you diabetes. Another study in Ontario said that grapefruit makes liver consume the over the top fat as opposed to putting away it. In this way, when you incorporate grapefruit in your eating regimen will you avoid diabetes as well as get in shape.

Do this:

Have a glass of grapefruit squeeze right in the morning to support your liver's fat smoldering limit.

On the off chance that conceivable, and on the off chance that you are edgy to get in shape, have grapefruit juice before each of your dinners.

Precautionary measure: If you are taking drugs, counsel your specialist before taking grapefruit.

Weight reduction home grown cures

Weight reduction home grown cures

8. Kelp Seaweed for Weight Loss

Furthermore, now a few privileged insights from Japan. Kelp ocean growth is widely utilized by Japanese as a part of their eating routine and the quality wellbeing parameters of this part of the world is not obscure. They are unquestionably slimmer individuals. So what makes kelp one of the best herbs for weight reduction! There are no less than two explanations behind this. In the first place, kelp is one of the wealthiest wellsprings of iodine. Iodine can keep your thyroid organ empowered so that your digestion system doesn't go slow. A supported digestion system implies your body goes through the calories quicker and better. Besides, ocean kelp has in it a compound called alginate. An exploration led at the Newcastle University found that alginate lessens the measure of fat your body retains. Amid the trial, the researchers utilized this ocean growth as a part of bread and reasoned that even a little measure of it diminished individuals' fat admission by around a third.

How to eat kelp for weight reduction?

While you can simply discover kelp supplements, its better to have them crude and natural. Incorporate kelp in an astypement of ways.

Use dried powdered kelp as flavoring for your dishes.

Make chopping so as to serve of mixed greens up crisp kelp ocean growth and blending it with different fixings such as cucumber, onion greens and so forth and decision of your plate of mixed greens dressing (low calorie dressing obviously!)

Add kelp to your soups to give it composition and some salty taste.

You can even utilize kelp to make your breads.

Safety measure: While kelp is useful for your thyroid and general wellbeing, inordinate utilization of this ocean growth can make your thyroid overactive prompting different wellbeing concerns. Likewise, those having kidney issues ought to counsel their specialists before fusing kelp into their eating routine. Pregnant ladies and nursing moms ought to take kelp under therapeutic supervision.

9. Thorny Pear for Weight Loss

Thorny pear is a desert flora plant whose more youthful adaptation is expended for the most part by Mexican and Mexican-Prickly pear cactus is customarily utilized as medication for diabetes, elevated cholesterol levels and certain different infections including obesity. With respect to weight reduction, thorny pear natural product is utilized which is now and then additionally called Indian fig. The American Journal of Clinical Nutrition has discovered high cell reinforcement levels in this natural product. At the point when your glucose levels are controlled, you have low levels of terrible cholesterol and get a decent supply of cancer prevention agents, you normally have a tendency to get more fit. Your enduring glucose levels don't make you want for sugary and boring nourishments. Certain cancer prevention agents too expand the rate of calorie blazing and fat oxidation. You can discover thorny pear natural products in the business sector that have as of now been cleared of their thistles. The entire natural product is high in fiber content which might offer you with weight reduction by making you some assistance with feeling full and moving your guts to lessen water maintenance. Be that as it may, you might likewise make thorny pear juice for your weight reduction diet.

How to make thorny pear juice?

Get this:

Thorny pear natural product 4

Do this:

Cut off both the finishes of thorny pear natural product. Presently additionally chop an opening down its body.

Peel off the skin of your leafy foods have the capacity to see the mash alongside numerous seeds.

Presently put the peeled thorny pears into your nourishment processor or utilize a blender to take out its juice.

Strain with the assistance of a sifter. Toss any seed on the off chance that they arrive in the juice.

Four natural products will give you around some juice.

Safety measure: If you are taking diabetes solutions, counsel your specialist first before having thorny pear. Pregnant and lactating moms ought to additionally converse with their specialist.

10. Gurmar Leaves for Weigh Loss

Gurmar leaves have been since a long time ago utilized by Ayurveda to treat different infections including diabetes, obesity, kidney stones and development of liver and spleen. It is one of the best digestive stimulant, diuretic and astringent herbs. "Gurmar" term of Hindi dialect signifies 'destroyer of sweetness.' When you bite the leaves of gurmar, you will lose your capacity to taste sweet for no less than 4 hours. This herb when taken inside equalizations your sugar levels furthermore enhances cholesterol and triglycerides levels. A few investigates have demonstrated gymnemic corrosive in these leaves is in charge of the said constructive outcomes. As this herb likewise lessens your sugar longings, this can be an awesome home grown solution for weight reduction.

How to assume gurmar for weight reduction?

Generally, 6-12 grams of powdered gurmar leaves are taken. This equivalents 1 – ½ to 3 teaspoons generally. On the other hand, on the off chance that you are a diabetic and are now taking meds, you should counsel your specialist before taking gurmar leaves for weight reduction. Its better to counsel an Ayurvedic expert or medicinal cultivator before you begin taking any herbs for weight reduction.

11. Coleus Forskohlii for Weigh Loss

Coleus forskohlii (Plectranthus barbatus), otherwise called Indian coleus, has a place with the mint group of herbs and is local to Southern Asia. It has been widely utilized as a part of Ayurvedic solution since antiquated times. The bases of coleus plant contain a compound known as forskolin. This segment offers your body some assistance with stimulating so as to burn fat thyroid capacity. Frskolin, truth be told, invigorates adenylate cyclase in thyroid layers which is in charge of controlling cells such as ATP and cAMP. ATP gives you vitality and cAMP is connected with adrenaline. When you take coleus forskohlii, you feel more lively and lesser hungry. It is more helpful for weight reduction in men as it additionally builds testosterone hormone. This herb diminishes both muscle to fat quotients and fat mass in men while expanding their incline body mass and bone mass. Numerous inquires about on men and ladies have demonstrated that ladies have a tendency to anticipate weight pick up and men have a tendency to get in shape with this herb coleus forskohlii.

How to take coleus forskohlii for weight reduction?

While coleus is utilized to make pickles and is a piece of vegan eating routine, you might jump at the chance to have this present herb's root extricate for weight reduction on the grounds that root is the part which is restoratively helpful for weight reduction.

Be that as it may, the entire base of the herb contains almost no measure of forskolin and may not give any restorative advantage. Get the one which contains 18 percent of forskolin. A run of the mill measurements of this herb incorporates 50 milligrams 2-3 times each day.

Precautionary measure: counsel your specialist before taking at all herbs for weight reduction, particularly in the event that you are under some medicine or are a pregnant or nursing mother.

Chapter 5

Simple exercises for weight loss

Peel off the pounds at most extreme velocity with this two-in-one cardio chiseling arrangement. Since you'll be performing quality moves at a heart-pumping pace, you can check cardio and resistance preparing off your schedule today!

How it functions: Do 1 set of every exercise all together without resting in the middle. Rehash the whole circuit 3 more times (4 times absolute).

You will require: Free weights

1. Plié Punch

Holding a couple dumbbells at hips with elbows behind body, stand with heels together, toes turned out around 45 degrees. Keeping heels squeezed together, expand left arm before shoulder, palm confronting down.

Step to one side and switch arms, squeezing right arm forward as left elbow twists, bending so as to bring down into a great plié position both knees out over toes, shoulders stacked over hips. Slide right heel once again into left as arms switch. That is one rep. Rehash until all reps are finished, rotating sides every time.

Sets: 4

Reps: 10

2. Pushed and Row

From a squat position, pivot forward from hips around 45 degrees, coming to dumbbells to floor. Twist elbows and push weights to either side of body, pressing shoulder bones down and together.

Crouch to floor and expand arms, squeezing dumbbells into ground straightforwardly beneath shoulders; hop feet once more into a full board position, attracting abs tight. Hop feet back in and come back to the beginning position; rehash.

Sets: 4

Reps: 10

3. Spiderman Pushup
Start in a full board position with hands marginally more extensive than shoulder-width separated, feet together. Lower into a pushup. Lift left knee into left arm (attempt to tap knee to elbow if conceivable). Come back to begin and rehash, exchanging legs on every rep.

Sets: 4

Reps: 10

4. Skull Crush Crunch
Get a couple of dumbbells and lie faceup with knees and hips twisted around 90 degrees. Twist elbows around 90 degrees so that the weights are in accordance with shoulders, palms confronting in.

Support abs in tight and smash up, lifting take and bears off the floor as arms reach out to roof (keep elbows lined up over shoulders). Gradually come back to begin and rehash.

Sets: 4

Reps: 15

5. Floating Lunge and Side Tap
Snatch a dumbbell in left hand and get into a low lurch position (attempt to bring back knee just a couple inches over the floor) with left leg forward, right arm stretched out up by ear, and left arm around side.

Support abs in tight and twist at the waist, coming to left hand to the floor, tapping the end of the dumbbell to the ground, admiring right hand. Come back to begin and rehash. Do all reps on the first side, then rehash on the other side to finish the set.

Sets: 4

Reps: 15 for each side

Any fruitful weight loss project is going to take you out of your usual range of familiarity, both in the rec center and in the kitchen. Powerful weight loss workouts are by and large vitality exhausting and physically and rationally burdened and best combined with a wholesome arrangement of assault that is loaded with sound, genuine nourishments (no prepared, fast food poop), which abandons you in a slight calorie shortage.

Enter the 6-Week Fat Blast.

To maximally diminish your muscle to fat quotients percent, you must begin in the kitchen. You might have heard the expression that abs are made in the kitchen, which is genuine - you can lose fat and not get a solitary weight or run a solitary step. Be that as it may, keeping in mind the end goal to assemble muscle, increment strong quality and cardiovascular wellness, you must hit the exercise center. Thus, to empower however much weight loss as could be expected, your system will comprise of 3 full body workouts for each week (substituting between Workout An and Workout B) with 2 days of cardio and 2 days off.

Cardio Workout 1

Begin with a 5-10 minute general cardiovascular warm up took after by 5-10 minute element drills (extends and skipping varieties).

Next, set up a treadmill to the maximal grade and at a rate you can sprint for 30-seconds. Set up a mat close to your treadmill with an exercise ball, a 50lb dumbbell and an abdominal muscle wheel.

Perform a 30-sec slope sprint and deliberately venture off the treadmill (keep it running).

Perform 30-sec Elbow Plank on the exercise ball.

Perform another 30-sec slope sprint.

Perform 30 reverse crunches while holding the dumbbell (which is set on the floor over your head).

Perform another 30-sec slope sprint.

Perform 30 abdominal muscle wheel rollouts from your knees.

Rehash this aggregate arrangement 8-10 times through.

Complete with a 5-10 minute general cardiovascular cool down.

Cardio Workout 2

Begin with a 5-10 minute general cardiovascular warm up took after by 5-10 minute element drills (extends and skipping varieties).

Next, set up a treadmill to the maximal grade and at a rate you can sprint for 60-seconds.

Perform a 60-sec slope sprint and precisely venture off the treadmill (keep it running).

Perform 20 stooping high link crunches.

Perform a rancher's convey with the heaviest dumbbells you can discover. Stroll beyond what many would consider possible before putting the dumbbells down.

Perform another 60-sec slope sprint.

Perform 20 horizontal pharmaceutical ball divider hurls per side.

Perform another rancher's convey pretty much as composed previously.

Rehash this aggregate grouping 6-8 times through.

Complete with a 5-10 minute general cardiovascular cool down.

Losing fat and bringing your muscle to fat quotients percent down is not as simple assignment. You're going to require an awesome bolster group to offer you some assistance with staying on track. Make a point to get enough quality rest every night to guarantee you can recuperation well in the middle of workouts – shoot for 7-9 hours for every night. Drink a lot of water separated for the duration of the day and plan solid snacks simply incase you're out and get hungry. Keep in mind, diet assumes all the more a part in weight loss than high power workouts. I'll end by rethinking a quote I read from wellness awesome Adam Bornstein: "Eat for the body you need, not for the body you right now have.

Chapter 6

Healthy lifestyle and weight loss

In our eat-and-run, huge segment measured society, keeping up a sound weight can be intense—and getting more fit, much harder. On the off chance that you've attempted and neglected to get thinner some time recently, you might trust that weight control plans don't work for you. You're likely right: most weight control plans don't work—in any event not in the long haul. On the other hand, there are a lot of little yet intense approaches to keep away from basic consuming less calories pitfalls, make enduring weight reduction progress, and add to a more advantageous association with nourishment.

The way to effective and weight reduction

Effectively dealing with your weight comes down to a straightforward mathematical statement: If you eat a greater number of calories than you blaze, you put on weight. What's more, on the off chance that you eat less calories than you blaze, you get in shape. Sounds simple, isn't that so? At that point why is getting thinner so hard?

Well for one, weight reduction isn't a direct occasion after some time. When you cut calories, you might drop a pound or so every week for the initial couple of weeks, for instance, and after that something changes. You eat the same number of calories however you lose less weight. And after that the following week you don't lose anything by any stretch of the imagination. That is on account of when you shed pounds you're losing water and incline tissue and also fat, your digestion system moderates, and your body changes in different ways. In this way, to keep dropping weight every week, you'll have to keep cutting calories.

Also, while basically a calorie is a calorie, your body responds contrastingly to diverse types of nourishment. So eating 100 calories of high fructose corn syrup, for instance, will differently affect your body than eating 100 calories of broccoli. The trap for supported weight reduction is to discard the nutritions that are pressed with calories yet don't make you feel full (like confection) and supplant them with nourishments that top you off without being stacked with calories (such as vegetables).

Thirdly, getting thinner in a sound, feasible manner frequently requires significant investment. It requires tolerance and responsibility. Great eating regimens might guarantee fast results yet will probably abandon you feeling grouchy and starving and losing more money than weight. At last, there are passionate parts of gobbling that can trip you up. A considerable lot of us don't generally eat essentially to fulfill hunger. We likewise swing to nourishment for solace or to calm anxiety—which can crash any weight reduction endeavors before they start.

The making so as to uplift news is that more astute decisions consistently, embracing sound way of life changes, and growing new dietary patterns, you'll not just get thinner and have the capacity to keep it off, you'll additionally enhance your standpoint and mind-set and have more vitality.

Preparing your mind to desire more advantageous nutrition

We aren't conceived with an inborn desiring for French fries and doughnuts or an abhorrence for broccoli and entire grains. This molding happens after some time as we're presented to more undesirable nutrition decisions. A late pilot learn at Tufts University, in any case, recommends that it's conceivable to reprogram your cerebrum's nutrition desires with the goal that you crave for more beneficial nourishments rather than unhealthy 'eating routine busters.' In the study, a little gathering of subjects selected in a behavioral weight administration program that underlines bit control and training to change dietary patterns. Following six months, mind examines uncovered expanded prize and happiness regarding sound, low-calorie nourishments, and a reduction in delight in unfortunate, higher-calorie nutritions.

While more research is should have been be indisputable, this is empowering news for anybody whose weight reduction endeavors have been undermined by horrible nourishment longings. You can figure out how to appreciate solid nourishment!

Beginning with solid weight reduction

While there is no "one size fits all" answer for lasting sound weight reduction, the accompanying rules are an extraordinary spot to begin:

Think way of life change, not transient eating regimen. Lasting weight reduction is not something that a "fast alter" eating routine can accomplish. Rather, consider weight reduction as a perpetual way of life change—a promise to supplant unhealthy nourishments with more advantageous, lower-calorie choices, diminish your bit sizes, and turn out to be more dynamic. Different famous eating regimens can kick off your weight reduction, however lasting changes in your way of life and nutrition decisions are what will work over the long haul.

Locate a cheering segment. Social backing implies a great deal. Programs like Jenny Craig and Weight Watchers use bunch backing to effect weight reduction and deep rooted adhering to a good diet. Search out backing—whether as family, companions, or a care group—to get the support you require.

Steady minded individuals will win in the end. Plan to lose one to two pounds a week to guarantee solid weight reduction. Getting in shape too quick can take a toll at the forefront of your thoughts and body, making you feel drowsy, depleted, and wiped out. When you drop a ton of weight rapidly, you're really losing generally water and muscle, as opposed to fat.

Set objectives to keep you propelled. Fleeting objectives, such as needing to fit into a two-piece for the mid year, more often than not don't function and also needing to feel more certain, support your inclination, or get to be more beneficial for your kids' sakes. Whenever dissatisfaction and enticement strike, focus on the numerous advantages you will procure from being more beneficial and leaner.

Use instruments that offer you some assistance with tracking your advancement. Keep a nutrition diary and measure yourself routinely, monitoring every pound and crawl you lose. By monitoring your weight reduction endeavors, you'll see the outcomes in highly contrasting, which will offer you some assistance with staying roused.

Where you convey your fat matters

The wellbeing dangers are more noteworthy on the off chance that you tend to bear your weight your belly, instead of your hips and thighs. A great deal of gut fat is put away far beneath the skin encompassing the stomach organs and liver, and is firmly connected to insulin resistance and diabetes. Calories got from fructose (found in sugary refreshments, for example, pop and handled nourishments like doughnuts, biscuits, and sweet) will probably add to this unsafe fat around your midsection. Curtailing sugary nourishments can mean a slimmer waistline and lower danger of malady.

Sound abstaining from food and weight reduction tip #1: Avoid basic pitfalls

It's continually enticing to search for easy routes however prevailing fashion diets or "snappy fix" pills and arranges just set you up for disappointment in light of the fact that:

You feel denied. Diets that cut out whole gatherings of nutrition, for example, carbs or fat, are basically unreasonable, also unfortunate. The key is control.

You get in shape, yet can't keep it off. Diets that extremely cut calories, limit certain nourishments, or depend on instant suppers may work in the transient yet do exclude an arrangement for keeping up your weight, so the pounds rapidly return.

After your eating regimen, you appear to put on weight all the more rapidly. When you radically limit your nourishment allow, your digestion system will briefly back off. When you begin eating ordinarily, you'll put on weight until your digestion system bobs back.

You break your eating regimen and feel excessively demoralized, making it impossible to attempt once more. At the point when weight control plans make you feel denied, it's anything but difficult to tumble off the wagon. Adhering to a good diet is about the 10,000 foot view. An infrequent binge spend won't slaughter your endeavors.

You understand lost when feasting. On the off chance that the nutrition served isn't on your particular eating routine arrangement, what would you be able to do?

The individual on the business lost 30 lbs. in two months—and you haven't. Diet organizations make a great deal of gaudy guarantees, and most are just implausible.

Low-sugar: Quick weight reduction however long haul wellbeing questions

Dr. Atkins' Diet Revolution propelled the low-starch diet furor, concentrating to a great extent on high-protein meats and full-fat dairy items, while banishing sugars, for example, bread, rice, and pasta. One mainstream stage of the low-carb eating routine is the South Beach diet, which additionally limits starches however supports more advantageous, unsaturated fats found in nuts and angle, and permits all the more entire grains, organic products, and vegetables.

The low-carb eating technique depends on the hypothesis that individuals who eat starches take in more calories and put on weight, while individuals on a high-fat eating routine eat less and shed pounds. Nonetheless, low-starch diets tend to shedding so as to bring about lack of hydration pounds as pee. The outcome is quick weight reduction, however following a couple of months, weight reduction has a tendency to moderate and turn around, pretty much as happens with different eating regimens.

The American Heart Association alerts individuals against the Atkins diet, on the grounds that it is too high in immersed fat and protein, which can be challenging for the heart, kidneys, and bones. The absence of products of the soil is additionally troubling, in light of the fact that these nutritions tend to bring down the danger of stroke, dementia, and certain diseases. Most specialists trust South Beach and other, less prohibitive low-starch diets offer a more sensible methodology.

Adjusted with authorization from Lose Weight and Keep It Off, an extraordinary wellbeing report distributed by Harvard Health Publications.

Solid abstaining from food and weight reduction tip #2: Put a stop to enthusiastic eating.

We don't generally eat just to fulfill hunger. On the off chance that we did, nobody would be overweight. Very regularly, we swing to nourishment for solace and stretch help. At the point when this happens, we every now and again pack on pounds.

Do you go after a nibble while sitting in front of the TV? Do you eat when you're focused or exhausted? When you're desolate? On the other hand to remunerate yourself? Perceiving your enthusiastic eating triggers can have all the effect in your weight reduction endeavors:

In the event that you eat when you're focused on, find more beneficial approaches to quiet yourself. Attempt exercise, yoga, contemplation, or absorbing a hot shower.

In the event that you eat when you're feeling low on vitality, find other mid-evening pick-me-ups. Have a go at strolling around the square, listening to empowering music, or taking a short rest.

In the event that you eat when you're desolate or exhausted, connect with others as opposed to going after the icebox. Call a companion who makes you snicker, take your canine for a walk, or go out in the open (to the library, shopping center, or stop—anyplace there's kin).

Solid abstaining from food and weight reduction tip #3: Tune in when you eat

We live in a quick paced world where eating has gotten to be thoughtless. We eat on the keep running, at our work area while we're working, and before the TV screen. The outcome is that we devour a great deal more than we require, frequently without acknowledging it.

Counter this propensity by honing "careful" eating: pay consideration on what you eat, appreciate every chomp, and pick nutritions that are both sustaining and agreeable.

Careful eating weight reduction tips

Focus while you're eating. Rather than chowing down thoughtlessly, relish the experience. Eat gradually, enjoying the scents and surfaces of your nourishment. In the event that your psyche meanders, delicately give back your thoughtfulness regarding your nutrition and how it tastes and feels in your mouth.

Maintain a strategic distance from diversions while eating. Do whatever it takes not to eat while working, staring at the TV, or driving. It's too simple to thoughtlessly gorge.

Have a go at blending things up to constrain yourself to concentrate on the experience of eating. Have a go at utilizing chopsticks as opposed to a fork, or utilize your utensils with your non-predominant hand.

Quit eating before you are full. It requires investment for the sign to achieve your cerebrum that you've had enough. Maintain a strategic distance from the allurement to clean your plate. Yes, there are youngsters starving in Africa, however your weight pick up won't help them.

Sound eating less carbs and weight reduction tip #4: Fill up with natural product, veggies, and fiber

To shed pounds, you need to eat less calories. In any case, that doesn't as a matter of course mean you need to eat less nourishment. You can top off while on an eating regimen, the length of you pick your nutritions shrewdly.

Fiber: the key to feeling fulfilled while getting in shape

High-fiber nutritions are higher in volume and take more time to process, which makes them filling. There's nothing enchantment about it, however the weight reduction results might appear like it.

High-fiber heavyweights include:

Foods grown from the ground – Enjoy entire organic products over the rainbow (strawberries, apples, oranges, berries, nectarines, plums), verdant servings of mixed greens, and green veggies of various types.

Beans – Select beans of any type (dark beans, lentils, split peas, pinto beans, chickpeas). Add them to soups, servings of mixed greens, and courses, or appreciate them as a generous dish all alone.

Entire grains – Try high-fiber oat, cereal, chestnut rice, entire wheat pasta, entire wheat or multigrain bread, and air-popped popcorn.

Concentrate on crisp products of the soil

Concentrate on foods grown from the ground

Tallying calories and measuring part sizes can rapidly get to be dull, however you needn't bother with a bookkeeping degree to appreciate crisp foods grown from the ground. It's by and large safe to eat as much as you need, at whatever point you need.

The high water and fiber content in most new foods grown from the ground makes them difficult to indulge. You'll feel full much sooner than you've tried too hard on the calories.

Eat vegetables crude or steamed, not fricasseed or breaded, and dress them with herbs and flavors or somewhat olive oil or cheddar for flavor.

Add nuts and cheddar to plates of mixed greens yet don't try too hard. Utilize low-fat serving of mixed greens dressings, for example, a vinaigrette made with olive oil.

Empty somewhat less oat into your morning dish to make space for a few blueberries, strawberries, or cut bananas. Regardless you'll appreciate a full bowl, however with a lower calorie number.

Swap out a percentage of the meat and cheddar in your sandwich with more advantageous veggie decisions like lettuce, tomatoes, sprouts, cucumbers, and avocado.

Rather than an unhealthy nibble, similar to chips and plunge, attempt infant carrots or celery with hummus.

Add more veggies to your most loved primary courses to make your dish "go" further. Indeed, even dishes, for example, pasta and blend fries can be eating routine cordial on the off chance that you utilize not so much noodles but rather more vegetables.

Take a stab at beginning your feast with a serving of mixed greens or soup to top you off, so you eat less of your entrée.

Sound counting calories and weight reduction tip #5: Indulge without overindulging

Make an effort not to think about specific nutritions as "beyond reach"

When you boycott certain nourishments, it is common to need those nutritions more, and after that vibe such as a disappointment in the event that you offer into allurement. Rather than denying yourself the undesirable nourishments you cherish, basically eat them less regularly.

On the off chance that you've ever ended up finishing a half quart of frozen yogurt or stuffing yourself with treats or chips in the wake of spending an entire day temperately eating servings of mixed greens, you know how prohibitive eating routine arranges normally end. Hardship diets set you up for disappointment: you starve yourself until you snap, and afterward you try too hard, counteracting all your past endeavors.

So as to effectively get more fit and keep it off, you have to figure out how to appreciate the nourishments you cherish without going over the edge. An eating routine that places all your most loved nutritions beyond reach won't work over the long haul. In the long run, you'll feel denied and will buckle. What's more, when you do, you likely won't stop at a sensible-sized bit.

Tips for getting a charge out of treats without indulging

Consolidate your treat with other sound nutritions. You can in any case make the most of your most loved fatty treat, whether it's frozen yogurt, chips, cake, or chocolate. The key is to eat a littler serving alongside a lower-calorie choice. For instance, add strawberries to your frozen yogurt or crunch on carrot and celery sticks alongside your chips and plunge. By heaping on the low-cal choice, you can eat an eating regimen cordial part of your most loved treat without feeling denied.

Plan your treats. Set up general times when you get the chance to enjoy your most loved nourishment. For instance, possibly you appreciate a little square of chocolate consistently after lunch, or a cut of cheesecake each Friday evening. Once you're molded to eat your treat at those times—and those times just—you'll quit fixating on them at different times.

Make your liberality less liberal. Discover approaches to decrease fat, sugar, or calories in your most loved treats and snacks. On the off chance that you do your own particular heating, cut back on sugar, compensating for it with additional cinnamon or vanilla concentrate. You can likewise take out or decrease fatty sides, as whipped cream, cheddar, plunge, and icing.

Draw in every one of your faculties—not only your taste sense. You can make nibble time more unique by lighting candles, playing calming music, or eating outside in a lovely setting. Get the most delight— and the most unwinding—out of your treat by cutting it into little pieces and taking as much time as necessary.

Solid consuming less calories and weight reduction tip #6: Take charge of your nutrition surroundings

Set yourself up for accomplishment by assuming responsibility of your nourishment surroundings: when you eat, the amount you eat, and what nutritions you make effortlessly accessible.

Eat early, weigh less. Early studies propose that devouring a greater amount of your day by day calories at breakfast and less at supper can offer you some assistance with dropping more pounds. Eating a bigger, sound breakfast can kick off your digestion system, stop you feeling hungry amid the day, and give you more opportunity to blaze off the calories.

Quick for 14 hours a day. Attempt to eat your last feast prior in the day and after that quick until breakfast the following morning. Contemplates recommend that this straightforward dietary modification—eating just when you're most dynamic and giving your digestive framework a long break every day—might help weight reduction.

Serve yourself littler bits. One simple approach to control segment size is by utilizing little plates, bowls, and mugs. This will make your segments seem bigger. Try not to eat out of substantial dishes or specifically from the nutrition compartment or bundle, which makes it hard to survey the amount you've eaten. Utilizing littler utensils, similar to a teaspoon rather than tablespoon, can moderate eating and offer you some assistance with feeling full sooner.

Arrangement your suppers and snacks early. You will be more disposed to eat with some restraint in the event that you have thoroughly considered solid suppers and snacks ahead of time. You can purchase or make your own little parcel snacks in plastic packs or holders. Eating on a timetable will likewise offer you some assistance with avoiding eating when you aren't genuinely ravenous.

Cook your own particular dinners. Cooking dinners at home permits you to control both part estimate and what goes into the nutrition. Eatery and bundled nourishments by and large contain significantly more sodium, fat, and calories than nutrition cooked at home—in addition to the bit sizes have a tendency to be bigger.

Try not to search for basic supplies when you're ravenous. Make a shopping list and stick to it. Be particularly watchful to maintain a strategic distance from fatty nibble and comfort nutritions.

Out of the picture, therefore irrelevant. Limit the measure of enticing nourishments you have at home. In the event that you impart a kitchen to non-weight watchers, store nibble nutritions and other fatty indulgences in cupboards or drawers out of your sight.

Sugar: The mystery diet saboteur

The vast majority of us expend more sugar than is solid, yet decreasing the measure of sweet and pastries you eat is just part of the arrangement. Sugar is likewise covered up in nourishments as astypeed as bread, canned soups and vegetables, pasta sauce, margarine, moment pureed potatoes, solidified meals, and ketchup. It's likewise in a considerable measure of nourishment.

Many prevailing fashion diets, get-healthy plans and inside and out tricks guarantee brisk and simple weight reduction. In any case, the establishment of fruitful weight reduction remains a solid, calorie-controlled eating regimen joined with exercise. For fruitful, long haul weight reduction, you should roll out lasting improvements in your way of life and wellbeing propensities.

How would you roll out those perpetual improvements? Consider after these six techniques for weight reduction achievement.

1. Make a pledge

Perpetual weight reduction requires significant investment and exertion — and a deep rooted duty. Ensure that you're prepared to roll out perpetual improvements and that you do as such for the right reasons.

To stay focused on your weight reduction, you should be engaged. It takes a great deal of mental and physical vitality to change your propensities. So as you're arranging new weight reduction related way of life changes, make an arrangement to address different burdens throughout your life in the first place, for example, monetary issues or relationship clashes. While these burdens might never leave totally, overseeing them better ought to enhance your capacity to concentrate on accomplishing a more advantageous way of life. At that point, once you're prepared to dispatch your weight reduction arrangement, set a begin date and after that — begin.

2. Locate your inward inspiration

Nobody else can make you get thinner. You should embrace eat less carbs and exercise changes to satisfy yourself. What's going to give you the blazing drive to adhere to your weight reduction arrangement?

Make a rundown of what's vital to you to stay inspired and centered, whether it's a forthcoming shoreline get-away or better general wellbeing. At that point figure out how to ensure that you can approach your motivational variables amid snippets of allurement. Maybe you need to present an empowering note on yourself on the storeroom entryway, for example.

While you need to assume liability for your own particular conduct for fruitful weight reduction, it has bolster — of the right kind. Pick individuals to bolster you who will energize you in positive routes, without disgrace, shame or attack. In a perfect world, find individuals who will listen to your worries and sentiments, invest energy practicing with you or making sound menus, and who will share the need you've put on building up a more advantageous way of life. Your care group can likewise offer responsibility, which can be a solid inspiration to adhere to your weight reduction objectives.

On the off chance that you like to keep your weight reduction arranges private, be responsible to yourself by having standard measure ins and recording your eating regimen and exercise progress in a diary.

3. Set practical objectives

It might appear glaringly evident to set reasonable weight reduction objectives. Be that as it may, do you truly know what's reasonable? Over the long haul, it's best to go for losing 1 to 2 pounds (0.5 to 1 kilogram) a week. By and large to lose 1 to 2 pounds a week, you have to smolder 500 to 1,000 calories more than you expend every day, through a lower calorie diet and normal exercise.

When you're setting objectives, consider both procedure and result objectives. "Exercise each day" is a sample of a procedure objective. "Lose 30 pounds" is a case of a result objective. It isn't crucial that you have a result objective, however you ought to set procedure objectives in light of the fact that changing your propensities is a key to weight reduction.

To keep your eating routine on track, attempt to get around eight hours of value rest a night.

4. Appreciate more advantageous nutritions

Embracing another eating style that advances weight reduction must incorporate bringing down your aggregate calorie consumption. However, diminishing calories need not mean surrendering taste, fulfillment or even simplicity of feast arrangement. One way you can eating so as to bring down your calorie admission is more plant-based nutritions — natural products, vegetables and entire grains. Take a stab at astypement to offer you some assistance with achieving your objectives without surrendering taste or nutrition.

Specifically, kick your weight reduction off by having a sound breakfast each day; eating no less than four servings of vegetables and three servings of organic products day by day; eating entire rather than refined grains; and utilizing solid fats, for example, olive oil, vegetable oils and nut spreads. Also, cut back on sugar, pick low-fat dairy items and keep meat utilization to a 3-ounce part (about the span of a deck of cards).

5. Get dynamic, stay dynamic

While you can get thinner without exercise, exercise in addition to calorie limitation can give you the weight reduction edge. Exercise can smolder off the overabundance calories you can't slice through eating routine alone. Exercise additionally offers various medical advantages, including boosting your mind-set, fortifying your cardiovascular framework and lessening your circulatory strain. Exercise can likewise help in keeping up weight reduction. Contemplates demonstrate that individuals who keep up their weight reduction over the long haul get consistent physical action.

What number of calories you smolder relies on upon the recurrence, length of time and force of your exercises. One of the most ideal approaches to lose muscle to fat quotients is through unfaltering vigorous exercise —, for example, energetic strolling — for no less than 30 minutes most days of the week.

Any additional development smolders calories, however. Consider ways you can build your physical action for the duration of the day in the event that you can't fit in formal exercise on a given day. For instance, make a few treks here and there stairs as opposed to utilizing the lift, or stop at the furthest end of the part when shopping.

It's insufficient to eat sound nutritions and exercise for just a couple of weeks or even months in the event that you need long haul, fruitful weight reduction. These propensities must turn into a lifestyle. Way of life changes begin with taking a legit take a gander at your eating designs and every day schedule.

In the wake of surveying your own difficulties to weight reduction, give working a shot a methodology to steadily change propensities and states of mind that have subverted your past endeavors. Also, you need to move past essentially perceiving your difficulties — you need to get ready for how you'll manage them in case you're going to succeed in shedding pounds for the last time.

You likely will have an incidental mishap. Be that as it may, rather than surrendering completely after a mishap, basically begin new the following day. Keep in mind that you're wanting to change your life. It won't happen at the same time. Adhere to your solid way of life and the outcomes will be justified, despite all all odds.

Chapter 7

Proper sleep and weight loss

Envision two ladies you know: One is your model of wellness achievement (She unmistakably knows how to thin down accurately and has the body to appear for it), and the other is the thing that you fear. This companion has her heart in the correct spot, yet regardless of how hard she functions, despite everything she battles with the procedure and doesn't have the body she needs. The alarming part is that when you converse with both, they share a typical methodology:

1. They eat dinners that emphasis on incline protein and vegetables.

2. They exercise no less than three times each week, concentrating on both weights and cardio.

3. They know which nourishments are genuinely sound and which they have to restrain—and they do.

Get More Workout Tips!

But then one companion—the person who keeps on battling—can't keep up her core interest. She experiences difficulty controlling her appetite, dependably hungers for desserts, and, in spite of her greatest endeavors in the rec center, she doesn't appear to accomplish the same results as another person taking after the same program.

The issue may appear glaringly evident at first. All things considered, one lady strays from her eating routine more than the other. What's more, if exercise "isn't working," it presumably implies she simply doesn't generally know how to prepare.

Possibly it's hereditary qualities. Perhaps she's languid or needs self discipline. Then again perhaps, eating regimen or exercise isn't the genuine issue.

Rest Controls Your Diet

The verbal confrontation about the most ideal approach to accomplish a solid weight dependably spins around eating and development. On the off chance that you need to look better, the most widely recognized proposal is "eat less and move all the more." But it isn't so much that straightforward, or even exact. At times you need to eat less and move all the more, however it appears to be difficult to do as such. What's more, there may be a justifiable reason: Between carrying on with your life, working, and working out, you're neglecting to rest enough. On the other hand possibly, all the more critically, you don't understand that rest is the way to being remunerated for your eating regimen and wellness endeavors. By Centers for Disease Control and Prevention, more than 35 percent of individuals are restless. What's more, when you consider that the measurement for obesity is about indistinguishable, it's anything but difficult to draw an obvious conclusion and find that the association is not a fortuitous event.

Not resting enough—under seven hours of rest for each night—can diminish and fix the advantages of counting calories, as per examination distributed in the Annals of Internal Medicine. In the study, health food nuts were put on diverse rest plans. At the point when their bodies got sufficient rest, half of the weight they lost was from fat. However when they cut back on rest, the measure of fat lost was sliced down the middle—despite the fact that they were on the same eating routine. Besides, felt essentially hungrier, were less fulfilled after suppers, and needed vitality to exercise. By and large, those on a restless eating routine encountered a 55 percent diminishment in weight loss contrasted with their very much refreshed partners.

Poor Sleep Changes Your Fat Cells

Consider the last time you had an awful night of rest. How could you have been able to you grope when you woke? Depleted. Stupified. Befuddled. Possibly somewhat cranky? It's not only your mind and body that vibe that way—your fat cells do as well. At the point when your body is restless, it experiences "metabolic languor." The term was authored by University of Chicago analysts who broke down what happened after only four days of poor rest—something that generally happens amid a bustling week. One late night at work prompts two late evenings at home, and before you know it, you're in rest obligation.

Be that as it may, it's only four evenings, so how terrible might it be able to be? You may have the capacity to adapt fine and dandy. All things considered, espresso does ponders. Yet, the hormones that control your fat cells don't feel the same way.

Inside only four days of lack of sleep, your body's capacity to appropriately utilize insulin (the expert stockpiling hormone) turns out to be totally upset. Truth be told, the University of Chicago scientists found that insulin affectability dropped by more than 30 percent.

Here's the reason that is awful: When your insulin is working admirably, fat cells expel fatty acids and lipids from your circulation system and avoid capacity. When you turn out to be more insulin safe, fats (lipids) flow in your blood and pump out more insulin. In the end this abundance insulin winds up putting away fat in all the wrong places, for example, tissues like your liver. Furthermore, this is precisely how you get to be fat and experience the ill effects of maladies such as diabetes.

Absence of Rest Makes You Crave Food

Numerous individuals trust that appetite is identified with resolve and figuring out how to control the call of your stomach, yet that is inaccurate. Appetite is controlled by two hormones: leptin and ghrelin.

Leptin is a hormone that is created in your fat cells. The less leptin you create, the more your stomach feels void. The more ghrelin you create, the more you empower hunger while additionally lessening the measure of calories you blaze (your digestion system) and expanding the sum fat you store. As it were, you have to control leptin and ghrelin to effectively shed pounds, yet lack of sleep makes that almost inconceivable. Research distributed in the Journal of Clinical Endocrinoloy and Metabolism observed that dozing under six hours triggers the territory of your cerebrum that builds your requirement for nourishment while likewise discouraging leptin and animating ghrelin.

On the off chance that that is insufficient, the researchers found precisely how rest loss makes an interior fight that makes it about difficult to get more fit. When you don't rest enough, your cortisol levels rise. This is the anxiety hormone that is much of the time connected with fat increase. Cortisol likewise initiates reward focuses in your cerebrum that make you need nourishment. In the meantime, the loss of rest causes your body to deliver more ghrelin. A mix of high ghrelin and cortisol close down the zones of your mind that abandon you feeling fulfilled after a feast, which means you feel hungry constantly—regardless of the possibility that you just ate a major supper.

What's more, it deteriorates.

Absence of rest additionally pushes you toward the nourishments you know you shouldn't eat. A study distributed in Nature Communications found that only one night of lack of sleep was sufficient to weaken movement in your frontal projection, which controls complex choice making.

Ever had a discussion like this?

"I truly shouldn't have that additional bit of cake... on the other hand, one cut won't generally hurt, right?"

Turns out, lack of sleep is similar to being plastered. You simply don't have the mental clarity to settle on great complex choices, particularly as to the nourishments you eat—or nutritions you need to maintain a strategic distance from. This isn't aided by the way that when you're overtired, you likewise have expanded movement in the amygdala, the prize district of your cerebrum. This is the reason lack of sleep wrecks all eating regimens; think about the amygdala as psyche control—it makes you hunger for unhealthy nourishments. Regularly you may have the capacity to battle off this longing, but since your isolated cortex (another part of your mind) is debilitated because of lack of sleep, you experience difficulty battling the desire and will probably enjoy all the wrong nourishments.

Furthermore, if all that wasn't sufficient, research distributed in Psychoneuroendocrinology found that lack of sleep makes you select more prominent bit sizes of all nourishments, further improving the probability of weight addition.

All that really matters: insufficient rest means you're generally ravenous, going after greater divides, and wanting each kind of nourishment that is terrible for you—and you don't have the best possible mind working to let yourself know, "No!"

Rest Sabotages Gym Time

Tragically the appalling effect spreads past eating routine and into your workouts. Regardless of what your wellness objectives are, having some muscle on your body is vital. Muscle is the foe of fat—it offers you some assistance with burning fat and stay youthful. Yet, rest (or deficiency in that department) is the foe of muscle. Researchers from Brazil found that rest obligation diminishes protein union (your body's capacity to make muscle), causes muscle loss, and can prompt a higher frequency of wounds.

Generally as critical, absence of rest makes it harder for your body to recuperate from exercise by backing off the creation of development hormone—your normal wellspring of against maturing and fat smoldering that likewise encourages recuperation. This happens in two distinct ways:

1. Poor rest implies less moderate wave rest, which is the point at which the most development hormone is discharged.

2. As already specified, a poor night of rest expands the anxiety hormone cortisol, which backs off the generation of development hormone. That implies that the officially decreased creation of development hormone because of absence of moderate wave rest is further lessened by more cortisol in your framework. It's an endless loop.

In case you're somebody who doesn't especially appreciate exercise, not organizing rest is similar to getting a physical look at with your father-in-law as the researching doctor: It will make something you don't especially appreciate verging on deplorable. When you're experiencing dozed obligation, all that you do feels additionally difficult, particularly your workouts.

The Better Health Secret: Prioritize Sleep

The association in the middle of rest and weight addition is difficult to disregard. Research distributed in the American Journal of Epidemiology found that ladies who are restless are a third more inclined to pick up 33 pounds throughout the following 16 years than the individuals who get only seven hours of rest for each night. What's more, with the greater part of the associations with obesity, diabetes, hypertension, heart disappointment, and subjective disappointment, the need to rest goes a long ways past simply looking better and getting results from your eating regimen and exercise endeavors.

While there's no hard number that applies to all individuals, a great general guideline is to get somewhere around seven and nine hours of rest for each night, and to ensure that one poor night of rest isn't caught up with a couple of something beyond. It won't appear like much, but rather it could have all the effect and mean more than little.

Chapter 8

Hormonal control and weight loss

Hormones are in charge of more than simply the periodic orgy. Their back and forth movement in your body control about each part of your weight, from when you get hungry to where you're well on the way to store fat. Indeed, even fat cells themselves discharge different hormones.

Something else you may not know: You can make these effective chemicals work for you. "Individuals have significantly more influence over their hormones than they might suspect they do," says Lena Edwards, M.D., chief of the Balance Health and Wellness Center in Lexington, Kentucky. These methodologies will offer you some assistance with taking charge more than five of the most compelling.

Promotion

Included Stories

Stunning San Francisco Luxury Properties You... Mansion Global

How One Woman Lost 40 Pounds of Fat and... Women's Health

Main 10 Oldest People In The World - Topz Share Topz Share

Step by step instructions to Speed Up Your Metabolism Women's Health

Lexus' new dashboard meter joins... Lexus Global

Prescribed by

Hormone: Leptin

One of the numerous hormones delivered by your fat cells is leptin, which assumes a part in ravenousness control. Research has found that abundance muscle to fat ratio ratios can bring about a condition known as leptin resistance, which implies your cerebrum isn't influenced by leptin despite the fact that your body contains more elevated amounts of it. In spite of the fact that it's still obscure precisely why this happens, one hypothesis is that as fat cells wrench out incendiary chemicals that square the activity of leptin, your body starts to believe it's starving. Clearly, that is not by any stretch of the imagination the case, yet to adjust for this apparent danger to survival, your digestion system backs off and your mind sends steady appetite signals with an end goal to compel you to eat, particularly fatty nutritions.

Equalization It Out: The uplifting news is that leptin resistance can be fought with eating routine and exercise. One thing that could: Try eating one measure of vegetables before 10 a.m. every day. Scott Isaacs, M.D., an endocrinologist in Atlanta and the creator of Beat Overeating Now! Take Control of Your Hunger Hormones to Lose Weight Fast, has found that individuals who take this guidance have a tendency to be less eager later in the day. Also, alongside satisfying fiber, vegetables contain fundamental cancer prevention agents and vitamins that have been appeared to decrease the aggravation that meddles with leptin, which thus increments fat blazing and lessen your longings.

Hormones: Cortisol and Serotonin

Ever ask why a chaotic day sends you plunging face-first into a pack of chips? That is the consequence of your adrenal organs discharging the anxiety hormone cortisol. That reaction, which is intended to give you a burst of vitality for battling or escaping, can frequently stay high because of supported anxiety, abandoning you longing for high-sugar or high-carb nourishments. There's even some confirmation that cortisol causes you to gather fat particularly in your stomach. Serotonin has the inverse impact: It quiets you down and is a characteristic ravenousness suppressant. Truth be told, the most up to date FDA-endorsed drug for weight reduction, Belviq, works by boosting the movement of serotonin in the mind.

Parity Them Out: To get the same impact without medications or sugary high-cal carbs, load up on folate-rich lentils, asparagus, and spinach. Your mind utilizes the B vitamins as a part of these nourishments to make serotonin. Getting enough rest helps as well; a study in the Journal of Clinical Neurology found that cortisol levels can twofold after a solitary dusk 'til dawn affair.

Hormone: Insulin

Each time you down a carb-loaded feast or sugary beverage that makes your glucose soar, your body reacts by discharging insulin, whose occupation it is to force additional glucose (sugar) from the circulatory system. Try too hard on pasta, bread, or desserts, and insulin can bring about those overabundance calories to be put away as fat, says Edwards. Sometimes, additional pounds can prompt insulin resistance, a condition in which cells turn out to be less receptive to the hormone, and to diabetes.

Parity It Out: You can control the measure of insulin your body produces and how well your cells react to it by decreasing nutritions that cause the greatest spikes in glucose. By study in Circulation, soda pops represent a full third of the included sugars in our weight control plans, so nixing them is an awesome begin. At that point exchange handled, refined carbs like white pasta and bread for entire grain adaptations, which contain fiber to moderate the retention of sugar into the circulation system, making for an all the more even-keeled insulin reaction. (Reward: The fiber will likewise offer you some assistance with feeling more full for less calories.) Spacing out your suppers and snacks so you're eating littler bits at more incessant interims for the duration of the day is another shrewd approach to keep up reliable levels of glucose and insulin, says Edwards.

Hormone: Irisin

A year ago, a study in the diary Nature reported the disclosure of an approach to make white fat—the kind we all know and loathe—carry on more such as cocoa fat, a kind that really copies calories. The key is presentation to a newfound hormone named irisin, which is delivered by muscle tissue and discharged amid exercise. The hormone likewise seems to diminish insulin resistance.

Parity It Out: Getting your sweat on is the main approach to increase irisin levels and, thusly, create more fat-blazing chestnut fat. In the Nature study, irisin levels multiplied following a 10-week stationary-bicycle preparing program that included four or five 20-to 35-minute sessions a week. Another, more subtle, strategy for expanding irisin is to alter your indoor regulator. Truly. Lower temperatures might make the white fat you have act like chestnut fat, moving your metabolic rate enough to bring about weight reduction, says Isaacs. One study found that when individuals burned through two hours in a 64°F room and intermittently plunged their feet into ice water, their cocoa fat smoldered 15 times a bigger number of calories than it did at room temperature—enough to wreck to nine pounds a year. (Better believe it, we're going to avoid the ice-water foot shower as well.)

Covered Chemicals

Hormones aren't made just by our bodies—they're surrounding us, sneaking in regular items. Look at three shocking spots where weight-pick up prompting hormones have as of late been found.

Scented Items

Numerous beauty care products, shampoos, and family unit cleaners contain chemicals called phthalates to help fragrances last. In any case, introduction to elevated amounts of phthalates has been connected to being overweight. Search for without phthalate on marks.

Canned Food

A few jars are lined with an estrogen-such as substance called bisphenol A (BPA). High-corrosive nourishments, for example, tomatoes, can make BPA filter into the can's substance. Search for without bpa jars or elective bundling.

Nonstick Cookware

Young ladies destined to ladies with the most abnormal amounts of perfluorooctanoic corrosive (PFOA) amid pregnancy were three times as liable to be overweight than those whose mothers had the least levels. PFOA is found in nonstick coatings, so utilize cast iron or stick.

For an immense number of us, the issue is rather about failing hormones. Exploration is as yet getting up to speed with this outlook change, which has yet to be thoroughly concentrated on. However, perceiving how this disclosure has helped my patients (and me) thin down and feel better gives me certainty that it's valid for most ladies why should attempting get in shape and can't. (Do you think wobbly hormones are bringing about your weight pick up? Discover how to control them and lose up to 15 pounds with The Hormone Reset Diet.) You definitely think about some weight-influencing hormone issues, similar to thyroid and insulin irregular characteristics. In any case, other, more inconspicuous ones could likewise be keeping you from the body you need. Science class, anybody?

1 Daily Teaspoon Of This Spice Could Help You... Prevention

·

What makes a vehicle emerge? See one... Lexus Global

The Diet Pill That's Scamming You Prevention

Prescribed by

How about we Stay In Touch

Agree to day by day wellbeing tips, in addition to elite offers.

You might unsubscribe whenever.

Your Privacy Rights | About Us

An excessive amount of Leptin Swells Your Appetite

Leptin swells your hankering.(Photograph by Stockfood)

I consider leptin the hormone that says, "Dear, put down the fork." Under typical circumstances, it's discharged from your fat cells and sets out in the blood to your mind, where it flags that you're full. In any case, leptin's respectable aim has been obstructed by our utilization of a kind of sugar called fructose, found in leafy foods nourishments alike. When you eat little measures of fructose, you're OK. Be that as it may, on the off chance that you eat more than the prescribed 5 day by day servings of organic product (which in late decades has been reproduced to contain more fructose than it used to) in addition to prepared nutritions with included sugar, your liver can't manage the fructose sufficiently quick to utilize it as fuel. Rather, your body begins changing over it into fats, sending them off into the circulation system as triglycerides and keeping them in the liver and somewhere else in your tummy. As more fructose is changed over to fat, your levels of leptin increment (in light of the fact that fat produces leptin). What's more, when you have a lot of any hormone coursing in your framework, your body gets to be impervious to its message. With leptin, that implies your mind begins to miss the sign that you're full. You keep on eating, and you continue putting on weight.

The alleged anxiety hormone cortisol can make a wide range of inconvenience for ladies who need to shed weight. At the point when cortisol rises, it energizes the transformation of glucose into fat for long haul stockpiling. Accumulating muscle to fat ratio ratios along these lines was a helpful survival adjustment for our precursors when they confronted unpleasant starvations. Less today. Clearly, lessening stress in your life will control this fat-putting away hormone, yet there's another extremely regular wellspring of the issue: day by day espresso, which lifts cortisol significantly, making your body to accumulate fat when you minimum need.

Crooked Estrogen Expands Your Fat Cells

Estrogen extends your fat cells.

In spite of the fact that estrogen is in charge of making ladies interestingly ladies, it's additionally the hormone that can be the most troublesome in the fat division. At ordinary levels, estrogen really keeps you incline by goosing the generation of insulin, a hormone that oversees glucose. At the point when estrogen gets misled, however, it transforms you into a weight-pick up machine.

Here's the manner by which: When you eat, your glucose rises. Like a bodyguard, insulin brings down it by escorting glucose into three better places in your body. At the point when insulin is in great working structure—not very high and not very low—it sends a little measure of glucose to your liver, an expansive add up to your muscles to use as fuel, and little to none to fat stockpiling. When you're sound and fit as a fiddle, your pancreas creates precisely the appropriate measure of insulin to have your glucose delicately rise and fall inside of a slender extent (fasting levels of 70 to 85 mg/dl). In any case, when your estrogen levels climb, the cells that create insulin get to be strained, and you can get to be insulin safe. That is when insulin begins to usher less glucose to the liver and muscles, raising the levels of sugar in your circulation system and eventually putting away the glucose as fat. Your fat tissue can extend by as much as four times to suit the capacity of glucose.

How do estrogen levels climb? Meat is one of the essential reasons. You take in significantly less fiber when you eat meat; research proposes that veggie lovers get more than twice as much fiber as omnivores. Since fiber offers us some assistance with staying normal, and we prepare overabundance estrogen through our waste, gobbling less fiber drives up our estrogen.

Meat additionally contains a kind of fat with its own estrogen issue. Ordinarily raised ranch creatures are over-burden with steroids, anti-toxins, and poisons from their food and the way they've been raised. When you eat them, those substances are discharged into your framework. They can carry on like estrogen in the body, adding to your over-burden.

Testosterone Slows Your Metabolism

Testosterone

You are gone up against with a shocking number of poisons every day, including pesticides, herbicides, hereditarily changed nourishments, and around six distinctive engineered hormones in meat. Poisons are prowling in face creams, professionally prescribed medications, prepared nutritions, your lipstick, the linings of fish jars, the flame retardant materials in love seats, and even the air you relax. The rundown goes on.

Numerous types of these poisons, for example, pesticides, plastics, and modern chemicals, act like estrogen when ingested in the body. Specialists trust that our expanding introduction to poisons clarifies why such a large number of young ladies are entering pubescence prior and prior and why numerous young men show female qualities, for example, creating bosoms. Xeno-estrogens, as these specific poisons are called, have been connected with a lifted danger of estrogen-driven illnesses like bosom and ovarian tumors and endometriosis.

5 Everyday Food Chemicals That Could Be Making You Gain Weight

This fake estrogen overpowers your body's testosterone—which is basic for hormone adjust—and adds to estrogen over-burden. Testosterone adds to muscle development, which thusly bolsters digestion system. What's more, as we definitely know, estrogen over-burden raises insulin obtuseness. The blend adds pounds to your casing: A study from Sweden distributed in the diary Chemosphere demonstrated that introduction to a specific type of pesticide called organochloride was connected to a weight addition of 9½ pounds more than 50 years.

Furthermore, that is only one kind of poison. Your danger of weight addition and infection from introduction to poisons might be more prominent than you understand. An overview by the CDC showed that 93% of the populace has quantifiable levels of bisphenol A (BPA), a substance found in store receipts and canned nutritions that disturbs estrogen, thyroid, and androgen hormones. Endocrine disruptors have been appeared to meddle with the generation, transportation, and digestion system of most hormones.

Presently you know the "whys" of your broken digestion system, the reasons general eating regimens don't address the main driver of your weight pick up. Hormones direct what your body does with nutrition. Fix your hormones and your body will thin down with no additional extra effort.

t's as old as time: The inclination to show signs of improvement shape in the New Year. Something around a crisp schedule year and a fresh start allures you to the exercise center bearing in mind the end goal of fresh starts, more advantageous living, and perhaps those washboard abs you've never entirely possessed the capacity to make happen.

In case you're similar to the a great many Americans who buy new rec center participations in January, you might be overflowing with inspiration right about now—which is extraordinary! Ride that flood of self discipline. However, it's not exactly what you eat and the amount you exercise that matters; understanding your hormones and how to function with them is an immense piece of weight reduction achievement.

Before you set out on your new year's weight reduction arrangement, become more acquainted with the three most persuasive hormones that are urgent to thinning down—and how to get them on your side.

Ghrelin

Created in your stomach, ghrelin is your craving hormone. On the off chance that you skirt a feast, your ghrelin levels rise and make you voracious, making it about outlandish for you to oppose the following nutrition thing you see. Hence, skipping breakfast to shave a few calories off the day is a major mix-up in case you're on the weight reduction train; ghrelin is high in the morning after you've fasted throughout the night, so you truly need to fuel yourself first thing to hold it within proper limits.

What's more, energizing with the right nourishment is pretty much as imperative as powering, period: A study distributed in the diary Clinical Science demonstrated that a high protein dinner brings down ghrelin levels altogether more than suppers high in fat and sugars. So concentrate on a high-protein breakfast, for example, casein and sans whey protein shakes, and veggie omelets. What's more, don't stop at breakfast—mean to get no less than 20 grams of protein at lunch and supper to keep ghrelin low after every dinner.

Leptin

Leptin is your useful sidekick on the weight reduction venture; you need no lack of this hormone if you will probably drop a gasp size or two. It's a ravenousness silencer, letting you know when to quit eating. Be that as it may, somewhat known certainty about leptin is that this current hormone's belongings in our bodies diminish with age. The more established we get, the more probable we are to have leptin resistance, which is the point at which our bodies don't react to leptin's signs (so your mind doesn't get the message to quit eating). To raise your levels of leptin and expand your affectability to this hormone, eat an eating regimen rich in omega-3 fatty acids and support your admission of nourishments that contain Eicosapentaenoic corrosive (EPA), which has been appeared to invigorate the creation of leptin. Attempt wild salmon, mackerel, and sardines. Absence of rest additionally brings down leptin and expands ghrelin, conveying on the desire to eat all the more, so make sure to get no less than seven and a half hours of shuteye.

Cortisol

Stress and cortisol go as an inseparable unit, and cortisol and gut fat go as an inseparable unit. At whatever time you're confronted with an upsetting circumstance, your body pumps out cortisol to meet the test. Cortisol urges your body to clutch instinctive fat—that extra tire around your waist—and it likewise drives you toward sweet and salty nutritions to control the strain you feel (they discharge delight impelling chemicals in the mind).

To neutralize cortisol's fat-putting away impacts, cut down on your espresso utilization and direct absolutely clear of it when you're feeling pushed. Caffeine taps your adrenal organs to discharge cortisol, which can be useful before a meeting or huge presentation since it hones your core interest. Be that as it may, when you blend caffeine with anxiety, your cortisol levels hop higher and stay high for more.

One study out of the University of Oklahoma demonstrated that expending 2 and a half to some espresso while under gentle anxiety made cortisol bounce 25 percent—and stay high for 3 hours. Another cortisol-bringing down tip: Make it a point to encompass yourself with constructive individuals who make you snicker! Essentially envisioning a giggle has been appeared to lower cortisol levels.

When you see how these three hormones work, you can make it simpler for your body to drop overabundance weight, and abruptly your weight reduction journey turns out to be less agonizing for you. Why starve on the off chance that it's simply going to raise your ghrelin levels and make it harder to oppose awful nutrition decisions? What's more, why not discover more opportunity for that clever companion on the off chance that she's a mystery weight reduction weapon?

As you push ahead with your more advantageous expectations this year, the most vital thing is that you trust you should look and feel better. You merit that leaner body, a more nutritious eating routine, a more advantageous heart, better vitality and the numerous different endowments that originate from making and regarding that dedication to yourself. Just cooperative attitude stream from it.

Chapter 9

Obesity and Diseases
Main 10 Obesity Diseases

More than 65 million grown-ups and 10 million youngsters experience the ill effects of obesity, considered one of the main sources of life-undermining ailments. Being extremely chubby can trade off your wellbeing, abbreviate your life, and even cause passing. In the event that you are overweight, the probabilities of creating coronary illness, diabetes, and hypertension increment altogether. Here are the main 10 obesity-related sicknesses.

1. **Hypertension** — High circulatory strain is the essential driver of death among Americans more established than 25. Around 75 million individuals experience the ill effects of hypertension or hypertension, which is a noteworthy danger element for coronary illness. Circulatory strain tends to increment with weight pick up and age. It is not known why obesity is a noteworthy reason for hypertension. On the other hand, research has demonstrated that corpulent patients showed an expansion in blood volume and blood vessel resistance. For individuals who are overweight and have hypertension, losing as meager as 8 pounds can diminish pulse to a protected level.

2. **Diabetes** Obesity is viewed as a standout amongst the most critical elements in the improvement of insulin resistance, and insulin resistance can prompt type 2 diabetes. By World Health Organization, more than 90 percent of diabetes patients worldwide have type 2 diabetes. Being overweight or stout adds to the improvement of diabetes by making cells more impervious to the impacts of insulin. A weight reduction of 15-20 pounds can offer you some assistance with decreasing your danger of creating type 2 diabetes. Perused: Exercising with Diabetes.

3. **Coronary illness** — According to the American Heart Association, obesity is a noteworthy danger element for creating coronary illness, which can prompt a heart assault or stroke. Individuals who are overweight are at a more serious danger of affliction a heart assault before the age of 45. Fat youths have a more prominent possibility of showing at least a bit of kindness assault before the age of 35 than non-stout young people. On the off chance that you are overweight, losing 10-15 pounds can lessen your danger of creating coronary illness. On the off chance that you exercise routinely, the danger of creating coronary illness falls considerably more. Perused: Benefits of Cardiovascular Exercise.

4. **Elevated Cholesterol levels** — High cholesterol is one of the main sources of heart assaults. Cholesterol is transported through your blood in two ways: the low –density lipoprotein (LDL), which transports cholesterol to the cells that need it, and the high-thickness lipoprotein (HDL), which is the sound cholesterol that lessens your danger for heart assault. Having high LDL levels raises your danger of having coronary illness by 20 percent. Losing 11-20 pounds can help you fundamentally lessen your cholesterol level.

5. **malignancy**

A study by the American Heart Association observed that being overweight expands your odds for creating malignancy by 50 percent. Ladies have a higher danger of creating malignancy in the event that they are more than 20 pounds overweight. General exercise and a weight reduction of as meager as 12 pounds can altogether diminishing the danger.

6. Impotence—
Being large can bring about changes in the hormonal levels of ladies, which can bring about ovarian disappointment. Ladies who are 15-25 pounds overweight are at a higher danger of misery from barrenness and ovarian tumor. Our bodies should be at a suitable weight to deliver the perfect measure of hormones and direct ovulation and feminine cycle. Try not to think men are resistant to barrenness. Overweight men have a more noteworthy shot of creating motility and a lower sperm number. Shedding 12-14 pounds can help you bring down the dangers.

7. Back Pain —
Obesity is one the contributing elements of back and joint agony. Unreasonable weight can make harm the most defenseless parts of the spine, which conveys the body's weight. When it needs to convey overabundance weight, the chances of anguish from a spinal harm or basic harm increment. Being overweight likewise raises the danger of creating osteoporosis, lower back agony, joint inflammation, and osteoarthritis. Losing 10-15 pounds can offer you some assistance with decreasing the danger of building up these issues.

8. Skin Infections —
Obese and overweight people might have skin that overlap over on itself. These wrinkled territories can get to be bothered from the rubbing and sweating, which can prompt skin diseases.

9. Ulcers —
According to a study by the National Institutes of Health (NIH), obesity can be a contributing element to the improvement of gastric ulcers. Gastric ulcers happen when there is an awkwardness between the measure of hydrochloric corrosive that is emitted and the catalyst pepsin. Overweight men are at a more serious danger of creating gastric ulcers than ladies. A weight reduction of as meager as 7 pounds can decrease the danger.

10. Gallstones —
Being extremely overweight expands the danger of creating gallstones, particularly in ladies. Gallstones are brought about when the liver discharges over the top measures of bile, which is put away in the gallbladder. Gallstones are more basic in more established ladies and those with a family history of gallstones. Losing 4-9 pounds diminishes the danger of creating gallstones. Moderate exercise additionally can bring warmth of temprament.

If you're hefty, will probably build up various possibly genuine wellbeing issues, including:

High triglycerides and low high-thickness lipoprotein (HDL) cholesterol

Type 2 diabetes

Hypertension

Metabolic disorder — a blend of high glucose, hypertension, high triglycerides and low HDL cholesterol

Coronary illness

Stroke

Tumor, including malignancy of the uterus, cervix, endometrium, ovaries, bosom, colon, rectum, throat, liver, gallbladder, pancreas, kidney and prostate

Breathing clutters, including rest apnea, a possibly genuine rest issue in which breathing over and again stops and begins

Gallbladder ailment

Gynecological issues, for example, barrenness and sporadic periods

Erectile brokenness and sexual wellbeing issues

Nonalcoholic fatty liver ailment, a condition in which fat develops in the liver and can bring about aggravation or scarring

Osteoarthritis

Personal satisfaction

When you're hefty, your general personal satisfaction might be lessened. You will most likely be unable to do things you used to do, for example, taking part in pleasant exercises. You might keep away from open spots. Large individuals might significantly experience separation.

Other weight-related issues that might influence your personal satisfaction include:

Wretchedness

Inability

Sexual issues

Disgrace and coerce

Social detachment

Lower work achievement.

Chapter 10

A step by step program to lose your weight

In case you're similar to numerous individuals, you have a requesting work, a family who needs you, and a ceaseless schedule. No big surprise you feel drained or discouraged, on edge or crabby. Alternately maybe you can't rest (despite the fact that you have no issue eating). Sex—or if nothing else great sex—is ancient history.

All are trademark side effects of endless anxiety. Stress actuates the battle or-flight reaction, the body's automatic reaction to a danger that makes our hearts pound and our breath abbreviate. Boss among the hormones discharged amid this reaction is the anxiety hormone cortisol.

Cortisol consequently kicks up your craving, provoking you to need to eat gigantic amounts as well as particularly to need desserts and straightforward sugars nutritions that make insulin levels spike and after that fall, which might abandon you feeling hungrier than any time in recent memory and eating once more, says Pamela Peeke, MD, collaborator clinical teacher of solution at the University of Maryland School of Medicine in Baltimore and creator of Fight Fat After Forty. "Stress fat" is likewise gathered in the last place you require it: somewhere down in your tummy.

To reset your inward stretch o-meter to ordinary levels, and maybe diminish stress-related hormonal desires, specialists prescribe the accompanying techniques:

Put enchantment photographs in your "anxiety zones." Clip to your visor a photograph from your commemoration excursion to Hawaii to quiet you when you're stuck in activity. Place in your work zone delightfully encircled photos of your youngsters.

Excerpted from The Hormone Connection by Gale Maleskey, Mary Kittel, and the editors of Prevention.

Talk some "quieting sense" into yourself. Quietly rehash a calming word or expression, for example, "peace," while taking moderate, full breaths through your nose. (Excessively occupied with, making it impossible to ruminate? Here's the way to sneak some mindulness in.)

Plan standard play periods into your arrangement book. Whether it's typeing out a 1,000-piece astound or sledding with your children, play occupies us from our stresses, giving an interim asylum from anxiety.

Giggle. In one study led at the Loma Linda University's Center for Neuroimmunology in California, a gathering of men who viewed a silly video were appeared to have 30% less cortisol in their blood and altogether lower levels of another anxiety hormone, epinephrine, amid and after the tape contrasted and a gathering that sat discreetly. Help up your drive with a tape or CD of your most loved entertainer or a silly book on tape. Look out for clever daily paper features or promotions. Also, obviously, watch motion pictures that make you chuckle.

Get a back rub. Profound weight rub animates the nerves that cause our levels of the anxiety hormones cortisol and epinephrine to go down, while the levels of two state of mind managing cerebrum chemicals that demonstration like the hormones serotonin and dopamine rise. This was valid in investigations of bosom growth patients, led at the Touch Research Institute at the University of Miami School of Medicine, and of ladies with fibromyalgia and unending fatigue disorder. Both gatherings reported lessened tension and wretchedness and enhanced disposition and personal satisfaction. Research has likewise demonstrated that people who give a back rub decrease their own levels of anxiety hormones.

Have intercourse. The more we do, the more endorphins our brains discharge. These "neuro-hormones"— chemicals discharged in the cerebrum amid exercise and, yes, after sex—are regular painkillers furthermore reduce tension. (On the off chance that your affection life needs a support, see 13 Tips For Seriously Better Sex.)

Week 2: Get a Good Night's Rest

Other than making you irritable, one hypothesis is that rest loss (under 8 hours of rest a night) might add to weight pick up by significantly upsetting the female hormones that control your dietary patterns and your digestion system.

In one little study, specialists in the University of Chicago's division of solution analyzed the hormone levels of 11 men while they got 8 hours of rest for a few evenings, trailed by a few evenings of a negligible 4 hours in bed. Amid the rest obligation arrange, the men's capacity to process glucose was impeded as much as a man with type 2 diabetes—showing that rest obligation could prompt insulin resistance, a condition a few specialists think supports obesity. In every one of the evenings that took after a restless night, the men additionally had reliably hoisted levels of cortisol, which urges your cells to store more fat, especially when matched with insulin resistance. Also the way that levels of thyroid hormone, the digestion system powerhouse, were brought down amid lack of sleep.

Whether you experience difficulty falling or staying unconscious, these master tips ought to offer assistance:

Get outside. The arrival of hormones in your mind is managed by the nerve driving forces sent by your retinas in light of light. At the end of the day, living by the world's common cycle of light and haziness keeps your serotonin and cortisol at their appropriate levels. Getting no less than 30 minutes of regular light a day resets our inward wake up timers, so we'll need to nod off at the ideal time, says Joyce Walsleben, PhD, executive of the Sleep Disorders Center at New York University in New York City and creator of A Woman's Guide to Sleep: Guaranteed Solutions for a Good Night's Rest.

Go out for a stroll. In one investigation of more than 700 individuals, the individuals who took every day strolls were 33% more averse to experience difficulty dozing until their typical wake-up time. The individuals who strolled energetically cut the danger of any rest issue considerably. Customary exercise eases stress furthermore raises body temperature, which primes us for sleep. (Perceive how to get the most out of your stroll with Power Walking.)

Decrease or take out stimulants, for example, jazzed espresso, tea, pop, chocolate, and nicotine before bed. Likewise, stay away from liquor, which is steadying yet disturbs rest.

Make your room dull. Obscurity fortifies the creation of melatonin, a light-delicate hormone delivered by the pineal organ, which is situated in the cerebrum. Some proof recommends that supplementing with this hormone can cure a sleeping disorder. (Take just briefly under the supervision of a proficient restorative specialist.) To control this hormone actually, put resources into thick, overwhelming window ornaments, or essentially wear an eye mask.[pagebreak]

Week 3: Eat Right

A sound eating routine can have a drastically beneficial outcome on female hormone levels. The fundamental arrangement? An eating regimen that is stacked with entire grains, crisp leafy foods, low-fat or without fat dairy items, and that contains less red meat and handled nourishments.

First and foremost, a high-fiber eating regimen can keep your glucose levels stable. Something else, nourishments made with refined grains, for example, white bread, white pasta, and white rice are processed rapidly and speeded into the circulation system as the body's essential wellspring of fuel: glucose. This quick breakdown triggers a surge of insulin, the hormone that ships the sugar into the cells. Presently, glucose levels drop sharply, which flags the adrenal organs to discharge more cortisol. By difference, beans, chestnut rice, and entire grain oats take any longer to process. So insulin levels rise continuously, glucose levels stay enduring, and cortisol levels don't soar.

Here are some different tips to trap your weight reduction hormones with nourishment:

Have "scaled down dinners." Instead of eating three major suppers a day-in addition to arbitrary snacks-eat five or six littler suppers separated out equitably for the duration of the day. Keep every dinner somewhere around 250 and 350 calories. "By eating littler yet more incessant dinners, with right extents of proteins, fats, and starches, you might be controlling your hormones for coming to the weight you need," says Geoffrey Redmond, MD, executive of the Hormone Center of New York in New York City and creator of The Good News about Women's Hormones.

Here are hypotheses concerning why scaled down suppers work:

Spreading little calorie loads over the span of a day might trigger development hormone, which keeps your body's digestion system proficient and smoldering calories.

The closer that one little feast is to the following, the less your glucose levels will take off, which implies lower insulin all the time.

Make breakfast an absolute necessity. It is the "single most noteworthy variable in keeping up part control and stable hormone levels for the duration of the day," says Dr. Redmond.

Start with a protein "canapé" 10 minutes before every dinner. It's conceivable that doing this sends your body the right flags not to gorge, since protein empowers the creation of the ravenousness directing hormones cholecystokinin and glucagon. Have string cheddar or a little modest bunch of nuts before you take a seat to eat.

Disregard without fat nourishments. Contrast names of without fat treats and their full-fat forms, and you're liable to find that, by and large, the calories of sans fat nutritions are as high or really higher. That is on account of sugar and other immediately processed straightforward starches are utilized to compensate for the fat-based fixings. Making so as to get your glucose off track can boomerang you hungrier in a short time.

Week 4: Exercise

Binding up your shoes is essentially an invitation to take action for the weight reduction hormones that invert fat capacity and check eating. "Your muscles are stacked with insulin receptors," says Christiane Northrup, MD, creator of Women's Bodies, Women's Wisdom and The Wisdom of Menopause. "The more bulk you have and the more warmth you produce from your muscles all the time, the all the more effectively you'll use insulin and smolder starches and muscle to fat quotients."

Strong confirmation moderate exercise—an energetic walk, a 45-minute "date" with the Nautilus machines—additionally triggers the arrival of "delight chemicals" known as endorphins. At long last, working up a decent sweat likewise actuates the "vibe great" neurotransmitters dopamine and serotonin, which lessen the indications of discouragement.

Made in the USA
Middletown, DE
22 March 2016